The Art of Helping Others

Being Around, Being There, Being Wise

Heather Smith and Mark K. Smith

Jessica Kingsley Publishers
London and Philadelphia

First published in 2008
by Jessica Kingsley Publishers
116 Pentonville Road
London N1 9JB, UK
and
400 Market Street, Suite 400
Philadelphia, PA 19106, USA

www.jkp.com

Library of Congress Cataloging in Publication Data
Smith, Heather.
The art of helping others : being around, being there, being wise / Heather Smith and Mark K. Smith.
p. cm.
Includes bibliographical references and index.
ISBN 978-1-84310-638-8 (pb : alk. paper) 1. Counseling. 2. Counselors. 3. Helping behavior. 4. Caring. I. Smith, Mark K. II. Title.
BF636.6.S65 2008
158'.3--dc22
2007044968

British Library Cataloguing in Publication Data
A CIP catalogue record for this book is available from the British Library

ISBN 978 1 84310 638 8

Printed and bound in Great Britain by
Athenaeum Press, Gateshead, Tyne and Wear

Heather Smith has worked in youth projects, a special school, a residential centre working with families where a child has a very serious or terminal illness, and a housing scheme for younger people. She has also worked in local projects with people who have, or had, difficulties around independent living and housing. Currently she is a lead tutor in a London further education college. She works both with students experiencing difficulties with studying and participation in college activities, and the staff who teach and support them.

Mark K. Smith has worked as a careers officer, youth and community worker and project worker. Now the Rank Research Fellow and Tutor at the YMCA George Williams College, London, he is working with the Rank Foundation on an evaluation of a large youth programme, and to develop new initiatives around community development and community leadership, and young carers. His publications include: *Creators not Consumers: Rediscovering Social Education* (1982), *Developing Youth Work* (1988), *Local Education: Conversation, Democracy and Learning* (1994), *Informal Education* (1996, 1999, 2005 with Tony Jeffs), and *Born and Bred: Leadership, Heart and Informal Education* (1999 with Michele Erina Doyle).

Contents

Acknowledgements

This book began with Parker J. Palmer. His explorations of the process of facilitating learning and the significance of the character and integrity of the teacher stimulated both of us to explore our own experiences – and those of the helpers we worked alongside. His ideas and example have been a constant inspiration and we have returned to them time and again in this book. We are indebted to him.

We also need to thank a large number of practitioners who have talked to us about what they were doing and feeling. This has included colleagues, friends and students. Their stories have both confirmed the significance of helpers rooted in local settings, and thrown considerable light on the processes involved and the meaning of the person of the helper. To them our thanks.

The book has been written with the support of the YMCA George Williams College, London, and the Rank Foundation. The book's support pages and materials appear courtesy of infed.org.

Finally, Heather would like to dedicate the book to mum and dad and those who have supported the work in progress! Mark would like to dedicate it with love to Michele, Michael and Matthew.

Introduction

Within any community there are special individuals to whom people turn for learning and counsel. Most of us can probably name at least one such person – someone who has made space for us to talk about our experiences, to deal with our feelings and to explore how we are to live our lives. We may describe these people as wise or caring. We may also recognize that it is something about the people they are, their integrity and authenticity, which allows them to touch our lives and to foster learning. Here we want to look at these qualities; what they mean for people who ask for help; and consider how those who are called to be around, wise and there for others may deepen the contribution they make.

To write this book we have drawn upon our own experiences and reflected on what we have seen others do. We have attended to the activities of some special people working within local settings and networks. This group includes social workers; youth workers and youth ministers; housing support and hostel workers; priests, nuns and lay workers within churches and religious groups; teachers, teaching assistants and learning mentors; and settlement, project and community workers. Many of these people are paid to be with others. All have some sort of recognized 'helping' or teaching role within a group or an organization. However, many of those we turn to for help and advice are neither paid nor have a formal role and title. They are part of, or linked to, the social networks to which we belong. We know them, for example, through family and friends, or meet them at work or through social activities. Often, they will not be fully aware of what they mean to people and the contribution they make. In this book we also look to their experiences and activities.

Our focus, in the main, is on being with, responding to and helping individuals around particular troubles and issues they face. For many, if not most people, the simple experience of someone being with them, listening to what they say and joining in conversation, can be affirming and healing.

But often people need to go beyond this. They need to go deeper: to explore experiences and situations, think about alternatives and possibilities, and consider how they might move forward. Conventionally, those who teach and counsel look to do this by setting up sessions – special time put aside to 'talk things through'. However, a significant amount of the exploration we are interested in here flows from helpers engaging in everyday actions such as cooking, talking over a cup of coffee or joining in with what a group is doing. Shared activity can often open the door for people to talk about things that are troubling them. They feel at ease or at least comfortable enough doing some other task to open up to another person. In these situations those called upon to teach and counsel have to be able to 'go with the flow', to respond by making space then and there for people to reflect on their experiences, attend to their feelings and spirit, and deepen understanding and commitment (Jeffs and Smith 2005). This may lead into setting up something more formal like a conversation or 'session' on another day; it may not. As people become known, they are also likely to be approached by those with whom they have had little or no previous contact.

There are all sorts of ways of naming these people. We chose to describe them as helpers. In some ways this underplays their significance and role. As givers of counsel, and explorers of experiences and feelings we might describe them as 'counsellors'. As facilitators of learning we could describe them as 'teachers' or 'masters'. After all, good teachers have the capacity to address 'the intellect, the imagination, the nervous system, the very inward of [their] listener[s]' (Steiner 2003, p.260). Another possibility is to talk about such people as 'informal educators' (Jeffs and Smith 2005) or 'local educators' (Smith 1994). The helping we explore here is characterized and driven by conversation; explores and enlarges experience; and takes place in a wide variety of settings (many not of the helper's making). However, describing the role exclusively in terms of counselling or teaching or educating narrows things down too much for us. Making sense of what these people are actually doing and expressing entails drawing upon various traditions of thinking and acting. This form of helping involves listening and exploring issues and problems with people; *and* teaching and giving advice; *and* providing direct assistance; *and* being seen as people of integrity.

The art of helping others

In our experience, people tend to use the words 'help' and 'helping' to refer to the process of assisting or coming to the aid of someone. When we help another person we make life easier or more possible for them in some way; we offer something that is useful. This can be quite mundane such as opening a door for someone who is laden with shopping. It might be something quite delicate, for example, being with a person as they try to come to terms with the death of their partner. The helping we are concerned with here may involve some direct, practical assistance – including providing people with something they need such as clothing or money. It also involves the complex process of being and working with someone around some difficult issue or question. Such helping is, at heart, a learning process – both for the helper and the helped. Done well it can be a space where people can come to know themselves and their situations better; to see possibilities and to believe that change is possible; and to take steps to overcome something that is troubling or facing them.

One of the problems with choosing 'helping' as the way of naming what we are exploring is that much of the literature does not really connect with the sorts of processes and concerns that we encounter among the helpers we have studied. Much of what is written is either skill-based and rather technical (see, for example, Carkoff 2000; Egan 2002; and Young 1998) or focused around dealing with particular issues (e.g. Briggs 2004). This is not to dismiss the significance of skill or knowledge about particular problems and issues, but rather to put it in its place. As David Brandon (1990) has argued in one of the few explorations of helping that does not fall into a focus on skilling, we have to attend strongly to the spirit in which helping is undertaken. 'The real kernel of all our help, that which renders it effective', he wrote, 'is compassion' (1990, p.6). It entails passion and commitment (Kottler 2000). Others have made the case for love (Brew 1957) and caring (Noddings 2002, 2005).

The helping we are concerned with flows in significant part from the person of the helper and their ability to reflect, make judgements and respond. It does not involve the simple application of knowledge and theory to situations. Rather it entails a particular sort of 'knowing'. One way of describing this is as 'artful doing' (Usher *et al.* 1997, p.143), another, 'artistry' (Schön 1983). As an art, helping exhibits sensitivity, judgement and the capacity to respond creatively in the here and now while holding on to the wider picture.

Elliot Eisner (2002) has argued that such an ability to reflect, imagine and respond involves developing 'the ideas, the sensibilities, the skills, and the imagination to create work that is well proportioned, skilfully executed, and imaginative, regardless of the domain in which an individual works'. He continues, 'The highest accolade we can confer upon someone is to say that he or she is an artist whether as a carpenter or a surgeon, a cook or an engineer, a physicist or a teacher'. Our focus here is, thus, on the person of the helper, their integrity and wisdom, and their ability to respond creatively and appropriately in their encounters with others.

The capacity to directly encounter and to help another is not easily developed (Rogers 1980, p.142). We have to be in touch with who we are and, at the same time, focus on the experiences, feelings and understandings of others. There is the constant danger of our projecting things onto them. We can easily fall into the trap of quickly categorizing people by the administrative frameworks we are often required to use, or by some experience in our own lives. Their reality and understanding might be quite different. What is more, our own craving for security, status and power can hinder growth, and undermine processes of self-help (Brandon 1990, p.6). As a result our attempts to 'help' can be more interfering than intervening. To encounter the other we have to be ready to meet them in some elemental way and be open to what they say and express in their lives.

Having and being

A good starting point for understanding all this is the distinction made by Erich Fromm (1979) and others between having and being. Fromm explores these as fundamental modes of existence, as two divergent ways of viewing ourselves and the world we live in. Having is concerned with owning, possessing and controlling. In it we want to 'make everybody and everything', including ourselves, our property (p.33). It therefore looks to objects and material possessions and, Fromm argues, is based on aggression and greed. In contrast, the being mode is rooted in love and is concerned with shared experience and productive activity. Rather than seeking to possess and control, in this mode we engage with the world. We do not impose ourselves on other beings nor interfere in their lives.

Instead, we act as whole beings so that all may flourish. To do this we place ourselves – who we truly are – in situations. We entertain ideas and experiences and allow them to touch us. Being is becoming. If we are open to others, and reflect on what they are saying, then we will change in some way as a result of our encounter with them – and so will others. Growth – of a person, a group or a community – is a possibility if we engage without a façade or front (Rogers 1980, ix and 115).

Fromm (1979, p.42) illuminates the differences between the two orientations by reflecting on their impact upon our experience of conversation:

> While the having persons rely on what they *have*, the being persons rely on the fact that they *are*, that they are alive and that something new will be born if only they have the courage to let go and respond. They become fully alive in the conversation because they do not stifle themselves by anxious concern with what they have. Their own aliveness is infectious and often helps the other person to transcend his or her egocentricity. Thus the conversation ceases to be an exchange of commodities (information, knowledge, status) and becomes a dialogue in which it does not matter any more who is right.

The work we explore here is based in being and presence. It flows from the 'aliveness' of the worker and their capacity to be themselves and part of conversations and encounters. Being able to respond to the other person, having a direct sense of how they might be feeling, we can join the play of thought and test out understandings. That playing and testing is, for the most part, best done face-to-face. It is not the same experience talking on the phone or exchanging e-mails. There is something very significant, we believe, about being in each other's presence. We can usually meet in a much fuller way.

Being around, being there, being wise

It may seem obvious, but for others to meet us as helpers, we have to be available. People must know who we are and where we are to be found. They also need to know what we may be able to offer. They also must feel able to approach us (or be open to our initiating contact). The sorts of encounters we are interested in here do not generally arise out of people making contact with some organization such as a counselling service (and being allocated a counsellor). Nor are they often the result of some formal referral. Rather these encounters are triggered by presence or a direct, personal approach. People know where the priest lives, for example, and knock on their door or call them on the phone. It is this direct availability in a neighbourhood, or in a particular setting such as a school, hostel or community centre that we talk about as 'being around'. In the latter settings it might involve us being in places where other activities are happening, perhaps in a coffee bar or in a common room. We may join in conversations or be there on some errand or duty such as running a fair-trade stall. Our presence and readiness to listen and talk means that it is possible, in theory at least, to respond to a person's question in time for it to matter. We are in the right place at the right time. Often it is a matter of 'catching the moment'; being able to pick up on something as it is said and to make space for exploration.

The presence of someone who is respected and who is known to care can also have an impact on people's experience of the settings where they are. On the surface we need not, as helpers, be doing very much other than welcoming or acknowledging people. The fact we are there alters things. We may be recognized as people with commitment and a history of contributing in an area. Our presence can thus help to stabilize and contain situations, and make things safe. McLaughlin, Irby and Langman (1994) have helpfully talked about this in the context of work with inner-city youth as the capacity to create urban sanctuaries. These are places of shelter and hope where young people are valued. They can be the buildings or institutions where helpers are based, or a temporary situation, for example, the section of a corridor where we are stood for a moment with a group. The presence of someone known as a helper in a setting can allow a group to gather, and conversation to flow.

As well as being around, we, as local helpers, are also able to 'be there' for people (Smith 1994; Jeffs and Smith 2005). By this we mean we are committed and ready to respond to the emergencies of life – little and large. We will sit with people as they try to make sense of the illness of a friend; accompany others as they deal with difficult situations such as appearing in court; and listen to the anger and distress of those who have found that their partners have walked out on them. At these points, people often are not able emotionally to 'think straight' about their situation. However, they may need to entertain some very frightening feelings. They also need to get through to the next day. For this they require the help of a particular kind of 'friend', someone who is constant, caring and has a sense of what might be going on for them. 'Being there' also involves a degree of practical assistance in dealing with the situations that people find themselves in. It might mean, for example, helping them to access and get something of what they need from distant and alienating systems such as those around income and housing support.

Last, as helpers we are called upon to be wise. We are expected to hold truth dearly, to be sincere and accurate (see Chapter 3). There is also, usually, an expectation that we have a good understanding of the subjects upon which we are consulted, and that we know something about the way of the world. We are also likely to be approached for learning and counsel if we are seen as people who have the ability to come to sound judgements, and to help others to see how they may act for the best in different situations, and how they should live their lives.

Working with

'Being there' is something of a 'holding operation' (Smith 1994, p.94). While it may involve deep-running emotions and commitment on the part of the teacher/worker, it may not be seen by them as 'working with' someone. 'Working with' is often reserved for describing more formal encounters where there is an explicit effort to help people attend to feelings, reflect on experiences, think about things, and make plans (p.95). This might involve putting aside a special time and agreeing a setting to talk things through (in much the same way as we might approach a counselling appointment or tutorial). Often it entails creating a moment for reflection and exploration then and there. It may be that we have to find a quiet place for such an interlude; or it could be that we alter the way we are with the other person and the focus of their conversation in the current setting. Whatever, the shift entails both parties recognizing and accepting that something called 'work' is going on. As helpers we are consciously and openly seeking to assist people to entertain, explore and develop with regard to some issue or situation. Furthermore, they accept this help and look to engage with the process. In this we both have to 'extend' ourselves; push the limits of thinking and feeling, assumptions and prejudices (Crosby 2001, p.55).

'Working with' is a special form of 'being with'. To engage with another's thoughts and feelings, and to attend to our own, we have to be in a certain frame of mind. We have to be open to what is being said, to listen for meaning. To work with others is, in essence, to engage in a conversation with them. We should not seek to act on the other person but join with them in a search for understanding and possibility. Attempting to impose some course of action or way of thinking on others, trying to win the argument, leads us from conversation into a form of the 'having' mode discussed above. It is, thus, important to stay in touch with whom we are, the values and ideas that inform us, and what we are feeling. This is also important for another reason. It is all too easy when listening to some story or issue to transfer our own meanings and emotions onto it, rather than allowing the truth to surface. We can be carried along on the emotion of the thing. If people are not in touch with who they are and what they think important then it is difficult to see how they can know another (Palmer 1998, p.2). Their sense and appreciation of others and the issues they face will be clouded and cluttered with debris.

'Working with' can also be seen as an exercise in moral philosophy (see Young 2006). Essentially, the helpers we are focusing on assist people to answer fundamental questions about themselves and the situations they face. At root these are concerned with how people should live their lives: what is the right way to act in this situation or that; of what does happiness consist for me and for others; how should I to relate to others; what sort of society should I be working for? In order to engage with this helpers need some appreciation of what might make for the good life; of what makes for human flourishing. They also need to be able to 'do philosophy': think in a rational and critical way about the world; the conduct of life; and the basis of belief. Furthermore, and crucially, they stand a much greater chance of being listened to and engaged with if they 'practise what they preach'.

> Everything depends on the teacher as a man, as a person. He educates from himself, from his virtues and faults, through personal example and according to circumstances and conditions. His task is to realize the truth in his personality and to convey this realization to the pupil. (Martin Buber reported in Hodes 1975, pp.146–7)

In other words, we have to struggle to live our lives as well as we can and be ourselves, if we are to connect and work with others.

Given all the above it is not surprising that working with people can often be 'a confusing, complex and demanding experience, both mentally and emotionally' (Crosby 2001, p.60). It is frequently the case, as a result, that many retreat from it. The cost – especially in terms of the uncertainties, confusions and feelings that truly attending to the other entails – can lead to all sorts of strategies to ensure that we are left untouched. Sometimes it is not easy to see. As Mary Crosby has commented, people's retreat may be concealed, even from themselves, 'by all kinds of activities which may look like "working with" people but are, perhaps, more a means of managing their own anxiety'. One of the classic moves here is to focus on technique and on more programmatic approaches. Rather than deal with the untidiness of people's lives and feelings, and to struggle with what might be appropriate responses – we simply take people through some predetermined assessment process and then into packaged programmes of talk and activity. At a stroke anxiety can be reduced. This outcome helps to explain the readiness of many teachers and workers to embrace government initiatives that require adherence to some curriculum or preset process.

On personal troubles and public issues

When working with individuals or groups we can easily end up working with people around the immediate issue or trouble. In C. Wright Mills' (1963, p.534) memorable words we can 'slip past structure to focus on isolated situations' and consider problems 'as problems of individuals'. We can confuse personal troubles with public issues.

> When, in a city of 100,000, only one man is unemployed, that is his personal trouble, and for its relief we properly look to the character of the man, his skills, and his immediate opportunities. But when in a nation of 50 million employees, 15 million men are unemployed, that is an issue, and we may not hope to find its solution within the range of opportunities open to any one individual. (Mills 1959, p.9)

Governments and corporations have a strong interest in seeking to divert and contain interest and activity around potentially destabilizing issues of this sort. Not unexpectedly, a lot of effort is put into defining and treating them as personal troubles. One result is the creation of programmes that look to bringing about individual change, for example, around eating habits, parenting, participation in education and training, and involvement in crime. Such initiatives do not usually, however, seek to encourage people to look behind the apparent 'trouble'; to question the economic and political forces that help create the problem in the first place. Nor do they facilitate people to 'take control of their moment' and to be defiant (Newman 2006, p.10). Instead, they are all too often staffed by what Mills (1963) called 'social pathologists' who frequently seem unable to rise above a view of people as cases to be managed; and who are paid to quieten dissent and the questioning of dominant systems.

If we can invite people to explore how economic and social forces structure their experiences and choices, and to think about their place in institutions, networks and neighbourhoods (see Bekerman, Burbules and Keller 2006), then there is, at least, the possibility of more rounded and appropriate learning and activity. We can look to the experience of the individual, the opportunities and constraints of the networks of which they are a part, and the limits of what might be achievable by a person on their own. This does mean examining 'who is trying to lay our futures out for us, who is telling us what we should and should not do, who is holding us back, and who is preventing us from acting effectively in our own and in others' interests' (Newman 2006, pp.58–9). It also entails putting a partic-ular stress upon working with individuals, groups and networks to deepen and extend their capacity to help. This area has been consistently underval-ued in state activity. Indeed, it is very difficult for the state and deeply professionalized forms of activity to have any direct involvement in this field without it tipping over into unwelcome forms of colonization (see, for example, Field 2003).

The book

In the first half of this book we explore what we view as some of the key characteristics of those who are able to respond to the experiences and feelings of others, and to help them to explore what has happened, deepen understanding and think about what might be done. They:

- appreciate what might be entailed in living life well and are called to do so
- know, and are able to be, themselves
- are concerned with truth and exploration

- put themselves in situations where they are able to relate well to others.

From there we go on to examine some key aspects of the process:

- being and acting so that people may explore, understand and commit

- sustaining and developing ourselves as practitioners

- creating space for more creative ways of being and acting within bureaucratic systems.

We argue strongly for ways of approaching helping that are rooted in care, commitment and calling. We also look to the needs of the whole person – and this, we believe, entails attending to physical, social, emotional and spiritual needs. Some reading this will dispute the inclusion of the last of these, others will, inevitably, be rooted in different religious traditions from ours. We have tried to write in an inclusive way but recognize there will be always be debates around the interpretations we make.

Our focus is on how we may cultivate our capacity to be with people; develop wisdom; and listen, speak and relate to others. It is this orientation and set of qualities that, we believe, many people search out when looking for someone to help them to reflect upon their situations, and to think about what they can do to make life better. This focus on the person of the helper – on being – and the spaces they create for truth to flourish takes us in a different direction from many books about helping, counselling and teaching. The central question is less 'what should I do?' than 'what sort of person should I be?' For those familiar with debates within moral philosophy this places our exploration within the tradition of virtue-based ethics rather than that of action-based ethics. This is not a focus that can be successfully approached via a step-by-step approach, nor through skills (at least not initially).

We also make the case for containing bureaucratic approaches that result in greater personal and structural enslavement for both helpers and the helped (Brandon 1990, p.111). This entails moving beyond many ways of working currently prized as 'professional' and embracing more local and improvisational helping.

In making these arguments we cannot draw upon great swathes of empirical data. Research into the experience and impact of helping relationships is difficult to conduct, and the data often impossible to interpret sensibly. It is hard to assess in any meaningful way for individuals what might have been the significant intervention or factor in the choices they make (Jeffs and Smith 2005, pp.87–90). We have relied heavily on reflection around, and exploration of, our own experience both as people who have needed help and been called upon to give it. We have also listened carefully to people who are called upon to be 'guides, philosophers and friends' to others.

We have tried to attend to the needs of those who have some recognition of their gifts as helpers, and who wish to develop their capacity to be and engage with others in ways that aid growth and flourishing. As a result, we offer some 'leading ideas'. With luck they may help people to make sense of their experiences and aspirations in this area. We hope that they will encourage reflection on how we, as helpers, can and should put happiness in its fullest sense at the centre of our activities; what it might mean for the ways in which people live their lives, and how we offer help to others.

Further reading and web support

- Brandon, D. (1990) *Zen in the Art of Helping*. London: Penguin Arkana (first published 1976 by Routledge & Kegan Paul). A landmark book, based in a strong appreciation of the relationship between personal troubles and public issues, and of the contribution that insights from Zen Buddhism could make to helping.

- Fromm, E. (2005) *To Have or To Be*. London: Continuum (first published 1976). This remains a rightly popular account of having and being. It calls upon us to resist dehumanization and to engage fully with life.

- Noddings, N. (2002) *Starting at Home: Caring and Social Policy*. Berkeley, CA: University of California Press. This book provides a good starting point for appreciating Noddings' work. It examines the nature of caring about and caring for, and sets it within more thinking around the nature of selfhood. It also has the bonus of some interesting explorations of different areas of social policy: education, housing and deviance.

For further discussion of the ideas explored in this introduction, suggestions for further reading and links to other sources, go to our support page at: www.infed.org/helping/intro.htm

1 Living Life Well

The helpers we are concerned with in this book work in a range of jobs and settings, and take on a myriad of roles. At first sight it can be difficult to see what they have in common. With job titles such as support worker, mentor, priest, community educator, project worker, guidance counsellor, nurse and youth worker it is likely that we will find some very different ways of working. However, when we begin to scratch the surface a number of strands emerge that run across these jobs. Within each, for example, there will be those of us who are required to 'deliver' some programme and achieve externally defined outcomes. This involves us in a technical exercise and is likely to dispose us to approaching those we are supposed to help in what we have seen Erich Fromm (1979) describe as a 'having' mode. We follow a formula or plan, and operate to correct procedures. Unfortunately, such a bureaucratic way of working has become an all too familiar feature of much contemporary schooling, social work and support work. In contrast, there will be others who approach their encounters with others with a more open commitment to fostering understanding and promoting well-being. This approach is more complex and personally demanding. We are asked to encounter and be with others, not act upon them. As a result, formulas and preset frameworks are next to useless. Instead we must make our way through a maze of conflicting notions about what is good, who it is good for, and how we discern the right course of action. At the same time we have to struggle to keep ourselves in the very state that we are promoting to others. It is this orientation, we believe, that lies at the heart of helping.

Acting with integrity, moral authority and authenticity is something that underpins the work we do as helpers. Without this we cannot do our job. As Parker J. Palmer (1998, p.10) has put it, 'good teaching cannot be reduced to technique; good teaching comes from the identity and integrity of the teacher'. Becoming someone that a community, a group of young people or an individual trusts, places a demand on us as practitioners to live life well. After all, how can we work with others around making life better without trying to do the best ourselves? Those who come to us for help will generally expect a high degree of consistency within and between both our professional and personal lives. Furthermore, questions around what it means to live life well often lie at the core of what people want to explore.

As a way into all this we want to suggest that living life well means living life in a way that promotes goodness in us, in others and in the environment. It may very well come back to the rule of 'do unto others what you would have them do to you'. It demands that we consciously engage in a way of being where we choose to do the right thing. To live life well means that we must 'preach' by actions rather than just words, and create living encounters and examples that others can experience and see. Nel Noddings (1992, p.90) has put this well with regard to bringing up children: 'To convey such messages authentically, we must talk with our children, live with them and show by our examples.'

In this chapter we will explore the notion of virtue, discussing what constitutes virtue, how is it achieved and maintained, and whether or not it is just accidental behaviour. We examine how we may live life well and care for others. We will explore the ideas of Eric Fromm in relation to self-love and then look at how we can extend this into caring for the needs of others. Finally we will look at the idea of connectedness and why we continue with practice that is often emotionally, spiritually and physically draining. For us the most helpful route to approaching these questions involves asking 'what kind of persons ought we to be?' rather than 'what should we do when confronted by choices involving right or wrong conduct?' In other words we have looked to virtue-based rather than action-based approaches to moral philosophy (see Haber 1993).

When looking at the ideas set out above, it is worth bearing in mind that it is our argument here that it is our character, identity and integrity – and the fact that we are around for others – that allow us to promote the idea of living life well to others. People do not seek counsel and learning from just anyone. As we pointed out in the introduction, people recognize that it is something about the people we are, our integrity and authenticity, and this allows us to touch others' lives and foster their learning. The idea of knowing who we are, and being that person, will be explored in much more depth in Chapter 2, but it is important to understand that it is who we are that animates our practice. We must be able to explore the notion of living life well in relation to how we live, not just how we promote it to others. We must be sure that we are able to practise what we preach.

What is virtue?

'Virtue' is a translation of the Greek word *aretē* meaning a kind of excellence – often of a functional kind. As Jonathan Haidt (2006, p.156) has noted, the *aretē* of a good knife is, thus, to cut well and 'the *aretē* of the eye is to see well'. However, the *aretē* of the human is much more difficult to agree. To begin, we can consider P. J. Chara Jnr's (1999) argument that virtues are 'principles of goodness and rightness in character and conduct that lead a person towards moral excellence and away from moral depravity' (cited in Roth, 1995). This notion is something that André Comte-Sponville (2001) has also supported in his popular exploration of virtues; he argues that a virtue is an excellence. For individuals to engage in virtue means they are engaging in excellence, aspiring to being virtuous is aspiring to be worthy of humanity (Comte-Sponville 2001, p.3). But what is 'worthy of humanity'?

When considering virtue we are inevitably drawn to the work of Aristotle. He looked less to principle and utility than character (Hursthouse 1999, pp.1–16). In his view, virtues are dispositions rather than skills; they are, as he put it, a kind of second nature. Virtue is not an emotion or faculty (the ability to feel the emotion) but a moral state. The virtue or excellence lies in people being in a moral state that enables them to perform their proper function well – to do the right thing rightly and to gain pleasure from that (Aristotle 1987, p.52). In this way a good life is one where you 'develop your strengths, realize your potential, and become what it is in your nature to become' (Haidt 2006, p.157). Individually speaking we all have the capacity of virtue, and whether we are able to be virtuous depends on our disposition. Aristotle offers this example:

> I call these moral states in respect of which we are well or ill-disposed towards the emotions, ill-disposed e.g. towards the passion of anger; if our anger be too violent or too feeble, and well disposed, if it be duly moderated. (Aristotle 1987, p.51)

It is our disposition or moral state that will inform whether we have been virtuous. For example, it is not because of our emotions that we are called good or evil, but because of how we react to our emotions. An angry person is not blamed because they feel anger, but rather for being angry in a certain way (Aristotle 1987, p.51). Such an emphasis upon character – and questions around what kind of person we should become – can seem strange. Much contemporary ethical enquiry focuses on actions – asking, as Haidt (2006, p.163) has commented, when a particular action is right or wrong. Thus, while virtues involve getting things right, just how we judge that, and what they might entail, is going to be a matter of continuous debate.

Many of the older accounts of virtue look to the practices and habits that display excellence of character. Christians (after Aquinas) define faith, hope and love (1 Corinthians 13:13) as virtues; Buddhists adhere to the six 'paramitas' of love, morality, patience, courage, meditation and knowledge. Confucian thought identifies charity, righteousness, propriety, wisdom and sincerity, and Aristotle adds temperance, justice, prudence and courage. It is important not to ignore the spiritual birthplace of the virtues. The very fact that a virtue is attached to religious thought and teaching indicates that the concern is not just with the practical ways in which we interact with others, but with how we can care for humanity on a higher level. Love, patience and wisdom all connect, for us, with the soul. Striving to be virtuous in these denotes a striving to connect with the 'indefinable essence of a person's spirit and being' (Whyte 1999) – and this goes a long way past simply engaging in a 'good' act.

Although we may be aware of what a virtue is, how do we achieve a state of virtuousness? Aristotle puts forward the notion that virtue is found at a point between excess and deficiency (1987, pp.55–6). The essence of any virtue lies in the balance, in the appropriateness of the action to the situation in hand, highlighting that the same action may not always be considered virtuous. As he put it, 'to experience these emotions at the right times and on the right occasions and towards the right persons and for the right causes and in the right manner is the mean or the supreme good which is characteristic of virtue' (Aristotle 1987, p.54). The virtue of love identified by Christianity can present an example. As children we are often free with our love and willing to love despite everything. At this stage love cannot be described as a virtue, because it is love in excess, but as we grow we begin to discriminate. Often adolescence and adulthood opens us up to being hurt by those we gave our love to, and so in order to protect ourselves we begin to strike a balance. We want to love, the lack of loving and being loved can create a void in the human spirit, but the balance needs to be sought. In order for love to be a virtue there needs to be discernment in how or whom we love. This illustrates Aristotle's argument about developing a way of being; we can be virtuous in love but not possess the virtue of love. This is true for any of the other virtues.

Virtue may indeed be about excellence of character, but striving for this 'excellence' in all we do can become a very arduous task and has the potential to leave us with feelings of failure, helplessness and frustration if we do not achieve the desired state. For virtue to have a practical application in the work we do and the way in which we live, for it to become more than a theorized notion, it is useful to explore being virtuous through our capacity to judge how to do 'the right thing in the place at the right time in the right way' (MacIntyre 1985, p.150).

Alasdair MacIntyre argues that a genuinely virtuous agent acts on the basis of true and rational judgement. By true, we mean that the agent makes an informed and committed choice to act. Doing the right thing demands of us that we deliberate and then both knowingly and consciously act in the interest of doing the right thing. But this 'consciously acting' does not always come with the luxury of time for deliberation. How many times have we been faced with a situation in the youth project, school or on the track that requires a decision there and then. When faced with the immediate we have to make a judgement call. But this does not mean that once we have made our decision about what was the right action and acted, that we will be left feeling virtuous. In making a decision about what was the right action, we can always be left with the question, 'what if?' After the event we can have the luxury of time and resources (usually other people) to reflect on whether we really did make the right choice. If we do decide that how we acted was not right, we then have to unravel the feelings we are left with. Rosalind Hursthouse describes these feelings as a 'remainder' (1999, p.47). As virtue centres on the person rather than the act, it is our handling of a situation that calls into question whether we acted virtuously rather than the actual act itself.

Focusing on the agent in isolation to the act and the context can cause problems. If we agree that living life well means the promotion of

goodness in us as well as in others, then we must also question the environment people place or find themselves in – and the actions they take. If we
ignore the bigger life picture of the agent, with regard to 'discrete actions
(telling a lie, having an abortion, giving to a beggar)' (Crisp and Slote
1997, p.3), then we are in danger of ignoring the effect they can have on
the agent's moral state. In the promotion of living life well, we must be
concerned with people's whole existence, rather than just how they react
to a situation.

The complication comes then for us as helpers, that the 'right thing' is
different in every situation. If we agree that the essence of virtue is found in
the balance between excess and deficiency, then we must accept that as virtuous practitioners or agents we will be constantly striving for that
virtuous state. Being able to identify and make a decision to do the right
thing in one instance does not mean that tomorrow it will be easy to make
a similar judgement. Genuine virtuousness is not accidental behaviour. Just
because someone acts with courage does not mean they are virtuous. It is
the deliberation and consciousness of the act that makes the individual virtuous in their courage. Consider the decisions we make, the people we are,
how we manage our practice; does it all happen by accident? Admittedly,
as helpers we usually have a gift for relating to others, but anything beyond
this basic 'like' for people is achieved through the decisions we make daily
on how to live and what is good and right.

Matt Ridley argues that virtues are about pro-social behaviour, and
engaging in virtuous acts enhances your reputation as a virtuous agent,
which in turn makes people more likely to trust you (1997, p.138). This is
where the connection between our 'professional' and 'private' worlds is
important. Being a helper in the community, in whatever capacity and with
whatever age group, demands consistency in our behaviour whether in or
out of work. This is something that we will explore in the next chapter
when looking at what it means to live authentically.

Flourishing and happiness

If we are to work with people so that they may grow we need to have some
idea about what might make for flourishing and happiness – what Aristotle
talked about as *eudaimonia*. For him, and us, this entails asking 'What
constitutes the good life for people?' The answers to this question

commonly appear in three forms: what people say makes them happy (the subjective); what we can measure 'objectively'; and what we think should be the case (the normative). It is important to appreciate what each can bring to our work as helpers.

Many contemporary discussions of happiness in everyday life are based upon a *subjective* reading of well-being. Researchers ask people about their current feelings; whether they are hopeful about the future and so on, and from this establish some measure of happiness in a particular time and place. This sort of approach is based on the belief that there is such a thing as 'feeling good' and 'feeling bad' – and that people can iden-tify and talk about it. Richard Layard (2005, pp.12–13) provides us with such a starting point:

> [B]y happiness I mean feeling good – enjoying life and wanting the feeling to be maintained. By unhappiness I mean feeling bad and wishing things were different. There are countless sources of happiness and countless sources of pain and misery. But all our experience has in it a dimension that corresponds to how good or bad we feel... [M]ost of us take a longish view. We accept the ups and downs and care mainly about our average happiness over a longish period of time.

Looking at the judgements that people make about situations and feelings, and the claims they make about their happiness, does seem to be an obvious starting point. When researchers talk to people about what makes them happy, and what causes them pain, a fairly consistent set of answers emerge. For example, Robert Lane's study (2000) showed strong links between subjective feelings of well-being and companionship (by which Lane meant family solidarity and friendship). We gain happiness through our relationships with other people: 'it is their affection or dislike, their good or bad opinion of us, their acceptance or rejection that most influences our moods (p.6). Lane found that once people rise above the poverty level happiness tends to lie in the quality of friendships and of family life. Increased income and the possession of more and more material goods have little impact on feelings of well-being. Other writers have used a range of published research and have come to broadly the same conclusions (see, for example, Offer 2006). According to Richard Layard (2005, pp.62–72), for example, seven factors stand out. These concern family relationships, financial situation, work, community and friends, health, personal freedom and personal values.

It is also possible that there are *objective* features of happiness. It can be argued that happiness is a tangible dimension of human experience – and that it can be measured (Layard 2005, p.224). Indeed, it has been increasingly possible to marshal a range of scientific evidence to support this view. Developments in brain and gene research, and more broadly in psychology and biology, have allowed us to talk with more certainty in this area (Lykken 1999; Martin 2005). We know, for example, that genetically we have a predisposition to a certain level of happiness (Shah and Marks 2004, p.5). How we feel does fluctuate, but it is possible to identify broad movements in our lives. These arise from the interaction of our genetic predispositions with our life circumstances, and the extent to which we set out to facilitate flourishing. However, we have only limited control over both subjective and objective factors. 'We do not choose the conditions into which we are born, and all sorts of contingencies plague human life' (Noddings 2003a, p.25). Furthermore, there is a limit to which we may 'act on' our genetic inheritance.

There is also a *normative* dimension to happiness. To appreciate this dimension, and to understand it in relation to education and welfare in the Western world, it is helpful to return to Aristotle. He and other classical thinkers like Plato and Socrates looked to claim happiness from contingency. That is, 'they wanted to define happiness in a way that makes it independent of health, wealth, and the ups and downs of everyday life' (Noddings 2003a, p.9). Happiness for them was something that referred to the whole life or the trajectory of a life. It was not episodic. In Aristotle's writings we can see two different conceptions. The first, 'comprehensive' view focused around eudaimonia and allowed for some contingencies. He recognized that wealth, health and friendship were significant but argued that the exercise of reason was 'the major component of happiness' (Noddings 2003a, p.10). His second, 'intellectualist' view was built around the notion that 'theoretical or contemplative thought is happiness'. This second understanding has fed into the view that there are higher and lower pleasures; that some forms of happiness are intrinsically better than others. While it is a matter of debate whether some forms of happiness are of themselves better than others, it does seem that people 'who achieve a sense of meaning in their lives are happier than those who live from one pleasure to another' (Layard 2005, p.22; see also Seligman 2003).

One of the striking features of political life and discussions around social and educational reform is the almost complete absence of any sensible conversation around well-being and what might make people happy. Instead much debate is formulated in terms of how education and social intervention might contribute to economic growth (which, as we have already seen, often has a negative impact on human flourishing) and upon achievement within the narrow boundaries of national curricula and the like. Sometimes we get some broad statements that can look like attention is being paid to questions of flourishing – such as in the much vaunted English initiative *Every Child Matters: Change for Children* (HM Government 2004). The government's aim, it was stated, was for every child, whatever their background or their circumstances, to have the support they need to: be healthy; stay safe; enjoy and achieve; make a positive contribution; and achieve economic well-being. The problem comes in both what is missed out or not made overt (such as the centrality of relationship, and omission of the transcendental), and the way in which aims are interpreted and prioritized. Often the devil is in the detail. When we come to look at how performance is actually measured a rather different set of concerns emerges (but more of this later).

If we truly place happiness at the centre of social and educational endeavour – both as something to be aimed at, and experienced in the process of learning and doing – then we enter a radically different debate. Education aimed at happiness, for example, cannot be achieved by simply teaching about happiness. We come to flourish in important ways through experiencing flourishing. This means cultivating spaces for learning and change where people can be happy. It also requires the involvement of facilitators and helpers who are happy in what they are doing and are seeking to live life as well as they can.

Caring for the whole person

To promote the well-being of others it is important to examine how we care for the whole person. As people we are multi-dimensional and multi-faceted. If we acknowledge this then our practice (and our being) must reflect this. Holistic care, or caring for the 'whole person', is concerned with the physical, emotional, intellectual and spiritual well-being both of ourselves and those we work with.

Care is described as the 'very Being of human life' by Martin Heidegger; it is the ultimate reality of life (cited in Noddings 1992, p.15). Nel Noddings argues that when we have a caring encounter, however large or small, we empty our soul of 'all its own contents in order to receive the other'. She goes on to describe this way of being as 'engrossment' (p.16). The nature of care requires attentiveness on behalf of the carer, and a willingness to receive by the cared for. Noddings argues that we all have the capacity to care, but that care is not a virtue. Although care may be seen as close to love, and referred to as an individual attribute as virtues are, it is in its essence about relationship. 'A caring relation is, in its most basic form', Noddings suggests, 'a connection or encounter between two human beings' (p.15). When we care for those we encounter, we must be attentive, and receive and acknowledge the way they need to be cared for. (We look at relationship in more detail in Chapter 3 and at caring in Chapter 4).

The physical well-being of others is usually an aspect of our practice that is tangible and easier to make decisions about. Health and safety guidelines are there to ensure that any trips or groups we organize are properly supervised and in safe surroundings, making sure that any risk is minimized. Child protection legislation and policies, for example, are intended to reduce the risk of harm to any child, giving us as helpers a reference point to ensure the safety of the children we encounter. Yet the emotional and spiritual side of our practice is seemingly more difficult to define and make decisions about. Each aspect of holistic care is inextricably linked, and often decisions about a person's safety and welfare are linked to a whole wealth of emotions, but emotional and spiritual care often have few guidelines to refer to.

As helpers, we need to appreciate that a key aspect of caring for others is caring for the self (see, for example, Seligman 2003). As we support the people we work alongside we must not underestimate – which we find is so often the case – the impact that their worries and concerns have on us as both practitioners and people. There is a widespread assumption that if you care about yourself or choose to put yourself first, that you are selfish (Fromm 1995, p.45). Yet if we don't care about ourselves, how are we able to promote care for others? Erich Fromm in *The Art of Loving* discusses various forms of love, but pays particular attention to the notion of 'self-love' (1995, pp.45–9). He argues that true self-love is not about narcissism, but about 'respect for one's own integrity and uniqueness, love for and understanding of one's own self' (p.46). He makes a link to the biblical idea of 'loving thy neighbour as thyself', and that we first need to understand and love ourselves before we can transfer this love and respect to others (p.46). If we have a love for humanity it must be acknowledged that we are part of it.

Jeff Kane also follows Fromm's line of thought. He highlights that the only way we are able to sustain the work we do is by taking care of ourselves (2003, p.169). If we agree that supporting and being alongside others necessarily 'injures' us (p.167), because it is our ability to 'feel' that informs our compassion, then as practitioners we need to acknowledge our own injuries. We need to tend to them as well as those of the people we care for. Recently one of us (Heather) was part of a team who gave emotional and practical support to families who had a child with a terminal or life-threatening illness. Her role was within a respite house where the family spends a few days in a home-from-home environment being looked after and cared for, allowing them to spend time together and giving each family member time to be himself or herself away from the pressures of the daily round. Although her practice was filled with fun and laughter, and many positive times of remission, there were also dark times when it seemed all hope had gone. At these times it was important that she was able to care for those who need it, but this was only possible if she acknowledged the impact her practice had on her, and tended to her grief as well. However, there had to be an appropriateness in how Heather dealt with her 'injuries'. It was not right for her to seek support from the people she was supporting; rather she turned to colleagues, her supervisor and her friends. By taking care of herself, she was able to continue caring for others.

Erich Fromm argues that genuine love is an expression of productiveness and it implies care, respect, responsibility and knowledge (1995, p.46). For Fromm it is a constant and active striving for the happiness and growth for an individual that is rooted in our own capacity to love. Jeff Kane (2003, p.138) once again follows up this idea and argues that caring for others involves us expanding our own selfhood; he calls this 'compassion's technology'. How do we use 'compassion's technology' in our practice? In working with others to promote their own emotional, social, spiritual and physical well-being, we as practitioners become, in crude terms, facilitators. It means decreasing the number of judgements we make without proper evidence and giving people room:

> Compassion means…opening doors rather than closing them; asking questions rather than giving answers. It means becoming aware of another person's situation and feelings. It involves listening with your whole being and giving, if you can, what is relevant and appropriate to the relationship without self-consciously measuring what it is. (Brandon 1990, p.49)

We take on the role of a sounding board – a person for a wealth of emotions to be directed at, a companion, a comfort, a guide; the list goes on. This makes it all the more difficult for us to define for the world exactly what it is we do. In examining this further we can look at the role of the mentor.

Within current policy initiatives both in the USA and the UK mentors are frequently assigned to those that society has deemed as dysfunctional in one area or another (Colley 2003; Rhodes 2002). This can be a positive assignment. It is often even more positive when people are free to choose 'mentors' – especially when they have developed a relationship with them through being with them perhaps as a member of a club or after-school programme (Hirsch 2005). The mentoring relationship can allow the mentee to explore situations, opinions and choices with someone who has no other attachment to them; the relationship is in the immediate. It gives scope for the mentee to establish a sense of his or her own self as an individual without being someone's son, daughter, brother or sister. This exploration is not exclusive to the mentoring relationship and features in many helping relationships. However, it is paramount that people are able to explore feelings and situations while feeling able to make mistakes. They need to know that their helper will still accept them and be there to work things through. However, this is not to say as helpers we become emotional punch bags and accepting of everything that happens within our practice. We need to expand our own selfhood to encounter others; know where we stand and yet be open to having our own preconceptions and opinions challenged; and reflect and change where appropriate.

As helpers we cannot pretend we do not have a history or views on what we consider to be a right way of living. However, we can allow our acceptance of others to be in the foreground. We may often be asked what we think or how we would act in a certain situation. This is where the challenge of working alongside others becomes apparent. It is easy to tell someone what we consider the right action to be, but we first need to ask 'who is it right for?' The ability to deflect direct questions about our opinions or ourselves is useful at times. Advice giving is often not appropriate and in the search for answers the onus needs to be put back on those we are working with. This is where the murkiness of emotional and spiritual support is most apparent. Practical advice giving on matters of process and systems, such as form filling, is helpful and of benefit. Advice on how someone should act emotionally or spiritually has the potential to go very wrong. For example, someone may approach us to discuss his or her relationship problems. He or she may tell us that they are unhappy and unfulfilled in their relationship and ask us what we would do in their situation. We may advise that they leave their partner, based on how we would act, given our own circumstances and way of life. As the individual trusts us, he or she may follow our advice but actually find him or herself in a worse situation, wishing they were back with their partner. They feel vulnerable and alone; who are they going to blame for their situation? Through not providing support that would allow the individual to decide their own course of action, the potential for further encounter and help has gone. As people who are sought for counsel, we must acknowledge (to ourselves and others) that we cannot provide answers, but that we are able to provide an environment and place of meeting where others can find their own answers. So how do we ensure that the 'right action' is promoted in such a subjective area?

In his work as a therapist, Carl Rogers (1961) promoted the idea of the client-centred approach and within the world of education a student-centred approach. The notion behind client-centred therapy is that each individual has within the ability to understand and to alter their own self-concept, beliefs and attitudes as well as their behaviour (1990, p.135). Rogers argued that these resources can be tapped into if an appropriate facilitative climate is established. This approach is not exclusive to a therapy relationship but rather applies whenever the development of a person is the goal. The ability to establish this type of relationship depends very much on us as practitioners being secure in who we are. When beginning a facilitative relationship as described by Rogers, he offers (p.121) that we first ask ourselves these questions: Am I able to enter someone else's world 'so sensitively that I can move about in it freely, without trampling on meanings which are precious to him'? Am I able to draw alongside another yet be 'strong enough as a person to be separate' and 'permit him his own separateness'?

The ability to care about others in a way that allows the individual to deem what is right for them requires an implicit trust in humanity and in a person's own ability to make decisions. As practitioners we can offer resources, experience and our own knowledge and expertise but must be willing to have them dismissed, and continue working with what the individual presents. Facilitative or helping relationships are about establishing an environment where the individual can take charge of themselves; if we provide this then we must accept what the individual decides.

If we examine this in relation to the previous question of how we promote the right action in the area of emotional and spiritual well-being, we must acknowledge that we cannot determine the right action for another. Rather we can establish a supportive environment, or meeting place, where an individual has the opportunity to explore what is the right action for him or herself and to consider their responsibilities to those around them.

Being connected

To live life well and develop our ability to care for the self and others, we must be able to connect with the people we encounter. A willingness to form and engage in 'helping' relationships demands a willingness to engage with humanity. Relationships, whether personal or professional, are often fraught with emotions and practical implications of being with another. Yet even at the height of this 'emotionally freighted interplay' (Storkey 1995) there is a deeper connection that keeps our engagement. At the heart of humanity, we believe, lies the soul – that of us that lies closest to God (or transcendental other) – a part of us that needs to be nourished and cared for. Through relating to and being with another person, we are able to build up a sense of belonging, both in our public and private domains – and, on occasions, to experience the transcendental.

Working with people can be uplifting, rewarding, comforting and hopeful, yet there are days when it is draining, exhausting and leaves us feeling claustrophobic. So what is it on those darker days that keeps us from walking away? Why do we continue to be a part of something that causes us distress? The simple answer is that we often stay because we care;

it is our ability to connect with the fragility of human nature that stops us from giving up. This connection often overrides what we are experiencing in the immediate (see Chapter 4).

Many of the relationships we form both personally and professionally are transient. Parker J. Palmer (1998, p.91), for example, highlights that most of us will achieve genuine intimacy with only a handful of people in a lifetime. In our practice it is not often that we are on intimate terms with the lives of the people we encounter. Because of this transience, we as practitioners need to have the ability to move on and develop new relationships each day. Through stripping away our preconceptions and judgements and turning as one human to another we can begin to sense what might be going on for others and appreciate the uniqueness of the individual. This gives us the freedom to have different encounters, by connecting with people through what they say, rather than basing assumptions on our own limited experience.

Look at our own practice: when we meet with someone do we really listen to what they say or are we making judgements because of what we know already based on context, history and environment? Through taking time to connect with the here and now of the individual it is possible to 'allow' someone to feel valued, listened to and understood. David Whyte in his discussion of the soul argues that 'a form of healing seems to take place when we find a truly sympathetic ear for our more difficult struggles'. He also suggests that 'just the opposite happens when we confide in someone who is simply not interested or is secretly scared to death of what we have just revealed' (Whyte 1999, p.53).

If we aspire to connect with humanity and have this as the basis of our practice, we need to put aside our fear of engaging with the rawness of life and instead embrace it. This is something that Palmer highlights. He argues that if we reclaim the connectedness of life we take away the fear of connecting (1998, p.58). The idea of connectedness is not about the specific relationships we have, rather it is concerned with a more basic relation to and empathy with human nature.

Conclusion

This chapter was aimed at exploring how we may live life well and whether our practice enables us to promote this to others. In exploring the idea of virtue we have looked at varying points of view but what has emerged is that being virtuous is about striving for excellence in character. It is not about having but rather being; it is concerned with our moral state and disposition. We have encountered writers such as Alasdair MacIntyre, Jonathan Haidt and Matt Ridley – all who have looked to Aristotle. Virtue is about consciously acting in the interests of doing the 'right' thing at the right time in the right way. Being virtuous, or at least striving to be, is not accidental behaviour.

We then introduced the idea of holistic care, identifying that we can only really care for another if we first take care of ourselves. Erich Fromm discussed the idea of self-love and we explored this in line with Jeff Kane's idea of expanding our selfhood to incorporate or encounter others. We then picked up on Carl Rogers' vision of client-centred therapy in order to discuss how we can promote the right thing for another person. What came out of this discussion was that if we are willing to walk alongside another and promote their well-being then we must also be willing to let them decide what is right for them.

Finally we touched on the notion of connectedness in relation to the idea that it is our deeper connection to humanity that keeps us sustained in the darker moments of our practice. However, although connecting with the rawness of life enables us to encounter others, it must be acknowledged that this is not always a salutary experience for either person. Engaging with reality stops us from becoming staid, and allows scope for true connection rather than that which is based on assumptions and preconceptions.

The notion of living life well, both striving for this for ourselves as well as furthering it in others, is something that goes hand in hand with the notion of authenticity. In the next chapter we will explore how we may achieve this in our practice and the implications it may have for us as both practitioners and people.

Further reading and web support

- Fromm, E. (1957) *The Art of Loving,* 1995 edn. London: Thorsons. Now marketed as a 'classic of personal development', this book is very different from most of the other books that inhabit the personal growth shelves in bookshops. Erich

Fromm's exploration of love is an exercise in social theory. He asks 'is love an art?', goes on to examine the theory of love, and then explores love and its disintegration in contemporary Western society. A final chapter examines the practice of love. While written from his distinctive humanistic perspective, the book looks to various religious sources to help make sense of love.

- Layard, R. (2006) *Happiness: Lessons from a New Science.* London: Penguin. This is a highly readable exploration of the nature of happiness and what makes us happy (and unhappy). In the process Layard undermines the supposed link between wealth and happiness and explores what can be done.

- Palmer, P.J. (1998) *The Courage to Teach: Exploring the Inner Landscape of a Teacher's Life.* San Francisco, CA: Jossey-Bass. This book is a modern classic. It draws together a number of the themes that Palmer develops elsewhere in his writing around the premise that good teaching (and helping) cannot be reduced to technique, but comes from the identity and integrity of the teacher.

For further discussion of the ideas explored in this chapter, suggestions for further reading and links to other sources, go to our support page at: www.infed.org/helping/living_life_well.htm

2 Knowing and Being Ourselves

As helpers we are often entrusted with people's ideas, thoughts and feelings, usually when they are feeling vulnerable, needing support or simply wanting someone to listen. This demands realness – in being who we say we are. Presenting a false image – a façade – can damage the potential for helping relationships, and can leave individuals feeling let down and mistrustful of others.

In this chapter we will explore the need for us as helpers to know who we are, and to be that person. We will look at how this notion relates to our practice alongside ideas of authenticity, integrity, character and the ability to be ourselves in what we do. Through the process of being with others, whether in good or bad times, we will be presented with a whole mixture of ideas and often feel challenged by them. It is important that as people who are trusted by others we are grounded in our own beliefs but are sensitive enough to have our belief system tested and even changed.

Knowing yourself

Consider how many times you have been asked, 'who are you', and then consider your answer. We expect you respond the same way we do with your name and possibly your job or reason for being where you are. But in relation to this chapter we need to explore this question in a different way. We need to look at who we really are, what has made us the people we are today. Each of us has a contrasting genetic inheritance, and a unique upbringing involving different significant adults and events. Yet for one reason or another we have found ourselves being sought for counsel and support.

In order to promote the well-being of others we must know and have an awareness of our own limitations, thoughts and feelings. In essence we must know ourselves. Parker J. Palmer (1998, p.2) picks out this theme when he argues that as a teacher, 'knowing myself is as crucial to teaching as knowing my students and my subject'. He comments that 'the more familiar we are with our inner terrain, the more surefooted our teaching – and living – becomes' (p.5).

> [K]nowing my students and my subject depends heavily on self-knowledge. When I do not know myself, I cannot know who my students are. I will see them through a glass darkly, in the shadows of my unexamined life – and when I cannot see them clearly, I cannot teach them well. When I do not know myself, I cannot know my subject – not at the deepest levels of embodied, personal meaning. I will know it only abstractly, from a distance, a congeries of concepts as far removed from the world as I am from personal truth. (Palmer 1998, p.2)

In this short paragraph, we find a clear rationale for attending to who we are, and what we are thinking and feeling. It is fairly obvious that self-knowledge is necessary if we are going to respond to people in ways that can further flourishing. Crucially, though, Palmer also makes the case for the significance of self-knowledge to subject knowledge and expertise. It is not surprising, therefore, that our development as people who can be turned to for counsel and learning is dependent upon us not only developing our ability to reflect on, and in, action (Schön 1983) but also to deepen our appreciation of ourselves.

Knowing is relational, we believe. It is the human way to seek relationship with another. We always talk about getting to 'know' someone, and holding someone at arm's length does not allow us to do this. To know ourselves we need to engage in a relationship with ourselves. We must embrace our fears, our hopes, our dreams, what makes us laugh and cry. There is a need to be in touch with what we feel and what makes us feel it. We need to be aware that how we see the world and experience it is often very different from the next person.

We respond to life's problems and circumstances quite differently from anyone else. This capacity is a reflection of our personal identity and allows us to experience life in a way that is distinct from others. It enables us to have our own unique take on the world. (Layder 2004, p.1)

This notion of knowing ourselves will be developed throughout this chapter when we explore ideas around selfhood, belief systems, authenticity and integrity. But what we must also consider is that in order for us to be able to further the well-being of others we must place ourselves in situations, agencies and environments where we can also flourish. This doesn't mean that where we find ourselves should be all hearts and flowers. Rather we should find ourselves in places where we are able to or at least have the scope to develop our ability to work with the challenges being presented. There is little or no point in placing ourselves in situations which do little more than break us. We need to be aware of how we cope with things, what we find difficult and what we are good at. For example, if we find adolescent behaviour difficult to understand and work with, there is no point gaining a job in a youth project. Equally, if we have strong anti-faith views there is no point placing ourselves in an agency where faith is fundamental to the ethos and everyday practice. This relates to the care of the self explored in Chapter 1, by knowing and acknowledging ourselves we are in a better position to create helping relationships with others.

Selfhood

There is a general tendency within Western culture to look at the individual as something that is quite separate and self-contained. There is a focus on the 'self' as 'I' rather than the self as part of a community, family or group. In this way of trying to understand the 'self' the body plays a crucial role. The skin becomes a boundary. Everything that happens outside the wall it forms becomes the *other* – the world outside; what is inside is *me* (Sampson 1993, p.34). Instead of considering how behaviours may affect others, taking into account the bigger picture, it becomes very much about the individual doing what is right for him- or herself, whilst paying little regard to what implications their actions may have outside of their 'self'.

This common Western view contrasts with a number of other cultures where individuals are viewed as more connected and part of a whole (see, for example, Marsella, Devos and Hsu 1985; Sorabji 2006; Taylor 1989).

Family, religion and groups play a large role in defining who individuals are, and set guidelines for behaviour and ways of living. There is an expectation that the individual will honour the role they have been given within a particular setup, acknowledging that their life is not simply about them. Another approach (which we take here) is to view the self as a relation constructed through encounter, dialogue and interaction (after George Herbert Mead and others). This notion flows from the idea that people's lives are 'characterized by the ongoing conversations and dialogues they carry out in the course of their everyday activities, and therefore that the most important thing about people is not what is contained within them, but what transpires between them' (Sampson 1993, p.20). Society and the individual are not viewed as separate entities. As Nel Noddings put it, 'We are influenced by others, and encounters with these others actually provide the building blocks of the self under construction' (Noddings 2002, p.112). More than this, if we are to develop the ability to care, we must allow ourselves 'to be affected by the needs and predicaments of others'.

How we view our own selfhood will affect how we as helpers interact and work with those who come to us for counsel and learning. If we view ourselves as separate and self-contained we may have a tendency to focus on what is going on inside. This may mean that when we work with individuals we may seek to develop the individual as autonomous and independent, and will focus on self-development. For those of us who focus on the notion of self as a part of a whole, the development of the group or community will become a focus. In respect of those of us who identify more with the view of the 'dialogical' self, the focus shifts from what is going on inside of the individuals to what is revealed and can be worked with in interaction. In other words, we look at individuals in relationship and seek to open up and deepen conversations and the conditions that underpin it.

We have all been brought up in different ways, experiencing different accounts of how the self operates. An awareness of how we view the self is important as it will have an impact on how we practise. But this appreciation is not sufficient when someone comes to us for help; there also needs to be an awareness of how they view the 'self' within their own lives. Understanding how the other person views the self can help us to approach how they view the world and to inform the way the discussions are formed and issues worked through.

Our character and belief systems

Each individual has his or her own personality. Our personalities are made up of qualities that make us unique but at the same time allow us to be compared to others. Because of the scope for comparison we, as helpers who are called upon to counsel and teach, have been marked out as different. We have a personality that draws others to us. In fact, we are our best tool. We have to 'use' who we are and how we relate to others as the basis of our practice. If we agree that relationships underpin what we do (see Chapter 3), then any material resources we tap into become secondary. Our primary and probably most vital resource is ourselves. Jeff Kane argues that, 'In this quintessentially low-tech effort, you yourself are the total technology' (2003, p.169).

There is a long tradition in the literature of counselling, youth work and informal education of exploring the character of the worker, identifying that it is the way we are that enables much of the work to take place (see, for example, Brew 1946). This supports the idea that we must allow ourselves to flourish and let our personality shine through into our work – not laid buried under the veneer of professionalism. We allow who we are to connect with others and lay foundations for future encounters and relationships, but this is not without its complications. As Bernard Davies and Alan Gibson (1967, p.175) put it in one of the classic works on social education, 'The contribution of the social educator must be made in personal terms: his personality is…the tool above all others which he will use in his practice.' Helping others allows few constants. Our daily practice environment may be the same, as may be the times we work, but the nature of the encounters we have depends very much on whom we meet, how they feel and how we feel at that given moment. The often-erratic nature of the work creates a need for us to know who we are and be ourselves within the given situation.

Davies and Gibson (1967) identify that, although our belief systems may not be overt in our practice, they will be present. Often what we think, feel and believe has had something to do with why we engage in our practice in the first place. They argue that it is our belief systems that enable us to act publicly for long, exhaustive, periods of time because they provide for us a firm foundation of personal assurance and support (1967, pp.177–80). This is why it is important to allow our personality and who we are into our daily practice. It is our firm grounding in who we are that allows us to be present in the uncertain and frightening worlds of others, and sustain that presence. However, Davies and Gibson also argue that there is relevance in separation of ourselves from our role in so far as we need to recognize that our practice is not an opportunity to canvass our own belief system (1967, pp.177–9). It is important to recognize that although our own thoughts, ideas and feelings will inform our responses to, and reactions within, the encounters we have, they shouldn't have free rein in influencing what takes place. We must develop the ability to use our characters as a tool but at the same time not allow who we are and our beliefs to dominate what happens within our practice. For example, a church worker may be approached by someone from a different faith who is having problems within their own religious organization. This is not an opportunity for the church worker to convert, rather a chance for the worker to support and sensitively explore and work with what the individual is experiencing. At the heart of each encounter should be the thought that we have been approached because we are thought of as someone who can be trusted and relied on. This image will be informed by our beliefs, but does not mean that we should promote them as the right way for another individual; with our support and understanding they must determine their own.

Using whom we are to build connections and relationships will affect our actions both in and outside of our practice. If we agree that who we are informs our practice, then with this comes a responsibility to be constant within it. There is a demand for us to be authentic and have integrity.

Authenticity

In his notion of client-centred therapy Carl Rogers argues that facilitators are more likely to be effective if they enter the relationships as themselves, meeting their client on a person-to-person basis.

> When the facilitator is a real person, being what she is, entering into a relationship with the learner without presenting a front or a façade, she is much more likely to be effective. This means that the feelings that she is experiencing are available to her, available to her awareness, that she is able to live these feelings, be them, and able to communicate them if appropriate. It means that she comes into a direct personal encounter with

the learner, meeting her on a person-to-person basis. It means that she is being herself, not denying herself. (Rogers 1990, p.306)

This not only creates the opportunity for a real encounter for the client, because they meet with the helper rather than a façade; but also it means that as the facilitator we are able to accept our feelings as our own, and this then goes some way to limiting the projection of our 'issues' on to the person we are meeting with.

The ability to be ourselves when others come to us seeking counsel and learning, whilst remaining aware that it is about them not us, is a complex notion and practice issue. There is a need to somehow achieve being authentic in who we are, yet not let our own enthusiasms take over or be forced on to the other. The notion of authenticity is concerned with something being exactly what it says it is; it is real, true and genuine (Taylor 1991). This can be easily understood in relation to using ourselves as a tool. If we present the idea that we are someone who can be trusted and relied on, then we need to be exactly that. This does not mean that we are there for others to the detriment of ourselves, but that if we choose to become a trusted member of the community then we have a responsibility to fulfil our role. As Derek Layder has argued, authenticity is about shedding pretences about yourself:

> It includes a lack of artifice and being transparently honest and sincere in your relationships (both with yourself and others). To be authentic is to be thoroughly genuine and trustworthy. This, of course, will feed into a firm sense of identity and integrity, because you are not trying to dupe others or trick yourself into thinking that you are something that you're not. (Layder 2004, pp.42–3)

For example, in their work with young people, guidance counsellors, youth workers and teachers will frequently present the image that they are there to listen should the young person wish to seek help from them. Consider if young people responded to this image yet found themselves meeting with someone very different, someone who had no time, empathy or inclination to listen or help. The potential damage is far-reaching. A young person may decide that all adults within the helping professions are like this – say one thing and mean another – and keep problems to themselves. This could lead to feelings of isolation and desperation. The experience of being let down may be told to their friends and thus the impact on the work of helpers is wider than that one encounter. This may sound melodramatic, but is actually very real and all too common in both our experiences. Consider the public image of social workers. Many do an amazing job yet we hear more (and publicly) about the few who don't, already causing damage to the relationships not yet formed.

However, this is not to say that as helpers we have to be on call 24 hours a day, and drop everything when approached. Instead it demands that we deal with each situation individually, assessing such things as urgency and need, and then sensitively decide a plan of action, either for a future meeting or an explanation as to why we can't respond there and then. It is better to be honest than risk losing the opportunity to meet with someone.

When thinking about authenticity we can become over-focused on our so-called 'inner life'. In part this can flow from a particular cultural under-standing and as we have seen there is a danger in many Western societies of taking on a very one-sided appreciation of what is meant by the self. Recent interest in authenticity, self-improvement and in discovering the 'real me' has tended to reflect a deeply individualistic turn. In the process it is easy to overlook the extent to which the stability of what we describe as our inner lives is achieved through social interaction and living in particu-lar social contexts (Williams 2003). Being authentic 'is not just a matter of concentrating on one's own self, but also involves deliberation about how one's commitments make a contribution to the good of the public world in which one is a participant' (Guignon 2004, p.163). This deliberation isn't just an individual matter either. Our claims have to make sense to others.

Integrity

Integrity plays a huge part in being a helper. We have already established that people may seek us out when they are feeling vulnerable, and because of this there is a responsibility for us to act with integrity when meeting with the feelings and emotions of another. To have integrity means to act in a way that adheres to moral principles, for example honesty. We have to handle people's emotions with sensitivity and care, and choose to act with good intention. Jeff Kane (2003, p.122) offers these thoughts: 'Words are so powerful, we must consider their possible effects carefully before we speak and then speak only with "TLC": truth, leanness and compassion.' This is not to say that we have to be perfect in our actions, but that we should be mindful of our compassion. Engaging mindfully means that compassion will become our natural style (Kane 2003, p.186).

Parker J. Palmer (1998) agrees that being who we are within our practice can only aid what we do, but acknowledges that this is not without its problems. He argues that although we can avoid stagnation in our work by being ourselves (p.48) this also makes us vulnerable. 'As we try to connect ourselves and our subjects with our students, we make ourselves, as well as our subjects, vulnerable to indifference, judgement, ridicule' (p.17). It is inevitable that being ourselves will affect us. Allowing ourselves to engage wholly means that there will be times when we are left feeling far from intact, yet this willingness to be touched can only deepen our understanding of human suffering; 'people who pretend invulnerability don't make good healers' (Kane 2003, p.180).

Being ourselves also brings with it having to accept and deal with personal criticism. There are ways to avoid this, and many of us do, by hiding behind our role, our qualifications and 'specialized knowledge', creating a professional rather than being a person. By doing this we are able to pass off any criticism as being about what we do, rather than who we are. However, if we want to follow through with the notion of being ourselves, being there and being around, we must accept that we will not always get it right, and that people will criticize us for this. It is what we do with the criticism that is important. We must be willing to learn by our mistakes and through what others have to say about us. This is not to say we should take all criticism to heart, but rather that we should be able to discern what we can take from it to enhance and further inform who we are and what we do.

So far we have looked at the idea of our belief systems, and the need to be authentic and act with integrity in order that those who seek us out can trust us. But what about those days when we simply cannot give, or find ourselves in a situation which totally goes against what we believe to be good and right. How do we stay true to who we are, both to ourselves and other people, whilst not compromising the relationships and encounters we have?

Being true to yourself

> I want to know if you can disappoint another to be true to yourself; if you can bear the accusation of betrayal and not betray your own soul; if you can be faithless and therefore trustworthy. (Oriah Mountain Dreamer 2000, p.58)

Oriah Mountain Dreamer asks whether we can be true to ourselves and bear being accused of breaking a promise. We all at some time within our practice and lives will find ourselves in situations we need to extricate ourselves from, even though we have promised support. The question that Oriah asks of us here is: what is the price if we don't leave; can we continue with our promise even if it betrays our own well-being? Healing and enabling exploration and learning is not meant to be sacrificial, we do not heal and help others and sacrifice ourselves in the process. There are times when we will need to say no, and admit that for one reason or another we cannot offer our help or time. We must acknowledge to ourselves and to others that this is okay. Jeff Kane describes a role-play session with some of his students where they were taking on the roles of doctors and patients. Many of the students vocalized the burden they felt at being a doctor:

> I felt like the patient dumped her whole life into my lap, and it was up to me to cure her or solve her problem. I wouldn't have felt 'professional' telling her that made me feel uncomfortable, or that I already had enough problems of my own. I felt like I had to look smart and competent no matter what. (Kane 2003, p.167)

As helpers we may also feel like this. When someone catches us on a bad day, when we are tired or are dealing with our own issues, the last thing we may want or need is someone asking us to listen to them. So what we do? Do we simply smile sweetly and reassuringly but not engage or do we continue engaging till we burn out? This is something that Jeff Kane (2003, p.183) acknowledges; he offers this piece of advice: 'Before you go to heal anyone, assess yourself. Do you feel up to it? If you don't, say so.'

However, this is often easier said than done. For those helpers for whom their practice is their work as well as part of their general life, it is not always viable to say that 'today I can't help', but it is important that we do. We can offer Heather's practice as an example. As already described, she was part of a respite team who supported families with children with life-threatening or terminal illnesses. Most days were filled with stories of hope and encounters with inspirational families and children. Yet there were days when it was hard to listen and support. She needed to be at work, so how could she manage her practice yet stay true to how she felt? The answer can be found in the ability to be honest with colleagues, being able to openly talk, laugh and cry about practice and find support within each other.

There are other ways in which we as helpers can discuss how we feel and find avenues of support. Many agencies and training programmes provide supervisors, field tutors and mentors. Supervision enables us as helpers to talk about our practice. Within these sessions we can identify how we feel, why we may feel this way and any practice issues that we may be facing. It gives us the opportunity to seek counsel. But the opportunity for us to seek counsel is not limited to this. Other avenues such as personal journals, practice journals and self-assessments provide us with the opportunity to articulate feelings, thoughts and processes we may be having or going through. It is essential that we ourselves keep talking.

But life is not just about work, and as helpers being sought for counsel it is not usually limited to our work environment. There will be friends and family who rely on our support and encouragement. Again we need to be honest with those who love us, admit that things are not all rosy and we can't offer our usual levels of support. This is probably the hardest lesson to learn. But being able to say you are finding it difficult to cope actually means you find a way to; in essence we have to be able to practise what we preach.

Another dimension of staying true to ourselves is the ability to extract ourselves from situations that compromise our integrity and beliefs. Part of being someone who is sought for learning and counsel is having a solid frame of reference that guides behaviour and action. If we engage in acts that portray our original claims as inauthentic, or portray us as immoral or people who cannot be trusted, our whole being as helpers is undermined. This is important to consider and highlights again the blurring of boundaries between our 'personal' and 'professional' lives. Bernard Davies and Alan Gibson argued that we should become 'literally "self-conscious"' (1967, p.175), not so that we are embarrassed of our actions, but so that we are aware of them and their implications. Being able to stand our ground in relation to what we believe and how we act is important not only for ourselves but also for those around us.

Being called to care

As we have seen, to truly be with another – to respond in ways that offer the hope of flourishing – entails being fully at home with who we are and what we are doing. It is an activity of the heart. We have to bring together our dispositions or habits on the one hand and emotions on the other so that we may act well (Gilman 2001, p.4; see also Halpin 2003). Without ability and commitment to give voice to these, hear truth and change, our capacity to engage with others will be limited. Yet it is one thing to know and be ourselves, quite another to offer to be with people and to help. We need to check whether we are in the right place, and doing the right thing. This is not some simple bureaucratic procedure. It is a matter of testing our calling (Palmer 2000).

The significance attached to calling and vocation (the Latin stem of vocation being *vocare*, meaning to call) has been diminished as occupational groups have taken on an emphasis upon technical skill and expertise; and upon adherence to policy (Collins 1991). Yet a concern with calling holds some hope for the helpers that are our focus here. As Michele Erina Doyle (1999) has argued, it honours the ethical base for practice, individual and group life, and emphasizes 'what we are, what we do and what we are to become'. All helpers are called and responded to. As she put it in relation to informal educators:

> Deny this and we undermine the relationship in which the work takes place, and the ability of people to invite us into conversations. Informal educators also call. They ask people to join with them in conversation. If no-one calls us, or responds to our call, we cannot be informal educators. (Doyle 1999, p.36)

In the light of this we need to take some care checking that helping is something we are called to.

The process of checking calling, and trying to discover and become 'who we are supposed to be, and what we are meant to do in the world' (Doyle 1999), is lifelong. It is easy to make mistakes and to follow false trails. Classically we can fall into the trap of trying to impose meaning on our experiences without letting them speak to us.

> Vocation does not mean a goal that I pursue. It means a calling that I hear. Before I can tell my life what I want to do with it, I must listen to my life telling me who I am. I must listen for the truths and values at the heart of

my own identity, not the standards by which I must live – but the standards by which I cannot help but live if I am living my own life. (Palmer 2000, pp.6–7)

If we do not listen for truths and values then we are likely to end up alienated from our relationships, our work and ourselves. There is also the danger of viewing our 'inner life' in isolation and failing to see how it is part of shared life. Calling has to be tested, it has to be experienced and recognized both by ourselves and by others.

Conclusion

The aim of this chapter was to look at how we can know ourselves and be that person. This opened up a wealth of discussion areas. We explored the concept of knowing and what this means both generally and with regards to ourselves. Drawing on the work of Parker J. Palmer we were able to see that knowing ourselves can enable us to know those we encounter. By being aware of who we are, we can be grounded in the teaching and counsel we offer.

We explored some different ways of viewing the self, establishing that how we view the self in relation to our own being will more than likely impact how we will interact with the self of others. This led us on to discuss the idea of our personality and belief systems, drawing on the ideas of Jeff Kane, Alan Gibson and Bernard Davies, and others. What came through at this point was that, for us to sustain our presence as helpers, we must have a firm grounding in who we are. Authenticity and integrity are fundamental to being around and being there for people. The very essence of our ability to do this lies in us being who we say we are. Because of the sensitive nature of being sought for counsel and learning, we must act in a way that is truthful and compassionate.

From there we went on to examine the importance of being true to ourselves, with regards to both recognizing our own needs and the ability to take ourselves out of situations that go against what we believe in. This also highlighted ways in which we can seek our own counsel when we are in need. Finally, we turned to calling – and the way in which our desire to help and educate others has to be tested.

The idea of exploring who we are and how this influences our practice is often criticized as being gratuitous reflection, and that more time should be spent on doing rather than thinking. Being sought for counsel and teaching does not exist independently of who we are. It is not a job to be 'done' but a way of being with people. The allowance and acceptance of separation between job and person creates room for bad practitioners. If a helper doesn't acknowledge himself or herself, the people they meet with and all the emotions that are wrapped up within that, how can they possibly offer counsel that has any depth, care or responsibility? As Carl Rogers (1990, p.120) put it:

> It is a real achievement when we can learn, even in certain relationships or at certain times in those relationships, that it is safe to care, that it is safe to relate to the other as a person.

Further reading and web support

- Layder, D. (2004) *Social and Personal Identity: Understanding Yourself.* London: Sage. This is an accessible introduction to understanding personal identity or self.

- Palmer, P.J. (2000) *Let Your Life Speak: Listening for the Voice of Vocation.* San Francisco, CA: Jossey-Bass. In this short, refreshing book, Palmer invites readers to attend to the 'inner teacher' and to follow its leadings.

- Kirschenbaum, H. and Henderson, V.L. (eds) (1990) *The Carl Rogers Reader.* London: Constable. The idea of genuineness or congruence is such a central feature of Carl Rogers' work that it is important to read him. Look particularly at his 1957 piece on the conditions of therapeutic personality change (reading 16), and his 1959 article on the person-centred framework (reading 17).

For further discussion of these ideas, suggestions for further reading and links to other sources, go to our support page at: www.infed.org/helping/knowing_and_being_ourselves.htm

3 Being Wise

Many of us have had our lives enriched by a relationship with someone we especially respect and talk about as being wise. She or he may have encouraged an interest or talent, been there for us in difficult times, or helped us to a deeper understanding of our lives. To do what they do they certainly have expertise – but often it is not just the knowledge they pass on or the advice they give that makes them special. Rather it is how they are with us, and we with them. We can feel valued and animated and, in turn, value them. Out of this meeting comes insight.

In this chapter we argue that helpers – those who are called upon to be, as Alexander Pope (1994) put it, 'guides, philosophers and friends' – are often not only trying to live life as well as they can and know themselves, but are also experienced as reflective, knowledgeable and discerning people. They are able to listen, talk and be with others in ways that allow experience, in that famous phrase of John Dewey's, to be emancipated and enlarged (1933, p.340). In other words, they are people of wisdom. They probably don't claim this for themselves. Wisdom is something that others associate with people rather than something they can claim for themselves. We earn or gain the description through what others experience of us. Moreover, if we have self-knowledge then we are likely to be only too aware of what we do not know and cannot do.

Sometimes people of wisdom are well known within local communities; they may even have some form of institutional status such as the priest or mentor. One us (Mark) was once taken to a Native American school in Minneapolis. There in a corridor was an older woman sitting with a group of children at her feet. The principal explained that she was the school's resident wise woman. Her job was to be around the school so that students could spend time in her company. She responded to what the children brought to her – difficulties they were having in their families or with their peers, questions about what was happening locally or in the news, pleasure in achieving a new skill. This woman, according to the principal, knew about the ways of local communities and understood human nature. However, she also appeared to have the capacity to be with people in a certain way. The way she carried herself, listened and asked questions allowed wisdom to flourish.

At a time when many professional helping relationships are increasingly governed by procedures and centrally determined outcomes, the idea that those who counsel and teach should be wise seems rather out of place. Within bureaucratic – and largely state-sponsored – systems the task of the 'helper' is often to assess and refer. The generally preferred judgement is technical and managerial. It is knowledge of the system rather than wisdom that is required by the role. Somewhere down the line those needing help may receive some 'package' of care, training and/or treatment. If they are lucky they might even come across someone, whilst being processed, who does give them time and space to talk about things in their own way and on their own terms. By way of contrast, if we look at helping relationships that are hunted out by those wanting assistance, then in our experience the wisdom of the helper is much more likely to be a key factor.

Wisdom and appreciating what living a good life might entail

When we describe another person as wise it can mean that we see them as learned or scholarly. In other words, we view them as having a deep understanding of some subject or knowing a great deal about the world. More especially, we may experience them as having a keen regard for truth and first principles. Alternatively, we may use the word to talk about someone who is able to come to sound judgements with regard to problems and situations. In this sense, wisdom is a capacity to judge well in matters such as the way we should live, how we should behave in different situations, and our goals in life. To be wise in this second sense does not mean that we have to be learned or scholarly – although it can certainly help. It does, however, entail knowing something about people and what makes them tick and about the world in general. This distinction is drawn from Aristotle. He differentiates between *Sophia* (philosophical wisdom) and *phronesis* (practical wisdom). As people who teach and counsel we need to open our hearts to both ways of knowing as each comes to inform the other – but more of this later. First, we need to return to a theme of the first chapter: appreciating what living the good life entails.

As soon as we use phrases like 'the capacity to judge well', we then have to address what might be 'right', 'just' or 'sound'. This inevitably leads us into questions about ends and means. It also brings us to ask questions about who might benefit from an action and who might lose – and how this relates to our own concern to be what we ought to be. Those of us who educate and counsel have a responsibility to consider the wider picture. We need to think about what might benefit the particular individual or group, and the impact of this on wider networks and communities as a whole. The judgements we are approaching are, thus, both political and moral. They necessitate asking what we should do in particular situations to make life better. They involve us in thinking about what is good. This takes us into the realm of moral wisdom – and the cultivation of it in ourselves and others. For the individual this entails deepening the human psychological capacity 'to judge soundly what we should do in matters seriously affecting the goodness of our life' (Kekes 1995, p.14). For communities it entails fostering spaces for reflection and engagement, and adopting policies that place happiness and the good at their core rather than material possession and economic growth.

It becomes clear then, that those of us called to be educators and sought for counsel in different communities need to have spent some time reflecting upon, and coming to some conclusions about, what might make for human flourishing and the good life. We also need to have developed a care about, and an ability to care for, others (Noddings 2003b). We suggest here that there are certain activities and behaviours that are characteristic of humans – and that it is possible to say whether these things are suited to them. Those that foster flourishing would then be constitutive of the good life (Brown 1986, p.135). There are also some fairly obvious candidates for inclusion on any list of 'goods', for example with regard to people having adequate means of subsistence; adequate food, clothing, shelter and so on; companionship and positive social relationships; and the ability to make a contribution through things like work and caring (Layard 2005). However, what this means for a particular individual or group varies. What might be right for one situation might not be for another. Such conceptions we have of the good life need to be carried as leading ideas, rather than as templates to be unthinkingly applied. We need to be open to other possibilities, to consider what might be for the good in this particular circumstance.

Being open to truth

We expect those called to be helpers to hold truth dearly. We anticipate that they will generally challenge falsehood, look beneath the surface, and be open to possibility. We associate truthfulness with their role. We expect them to display the 'two basic virtues of truth': sincerity and accuracy (Williams 2003, p.11). This may well, in part, be linked historically to religious expectations. In Christian traditions, for example, bearing false witness would usually be seen as undermining the foundations of God's covenant. However, there are purely secular reasons for having a regard for truth. Without it, economic and social relationships would be difficult to sustain as there would be little reason to trust the other (Beem 1999; Putnam 2000). There would also be little possibility of the advancement of knowledge. It would be impossible to evaluate one claim against another. We should expect helpers of the kind we are discussing here, as Bernard Williams (2003, p.11) has put it, to do their best to acquire 'true beliefs' and that what they say actually reveals what they believe. Their authority, he continues, 'must be rooted in their truthfulness in both these respects: they take care, and they do not lie'. This can, however, come into conflict with other 'goods'. Human flourishing, for example, might be served in certain instances by not saying what we believe to be true (see Bok 1999 and Chapter 7).

Some of the difficulties we can experience here relate to debates about the nature of truth. For many people, as for Aristotle and Plato, truth is 'correspondence' with the facts; it is agreement with reality (Kirkman 1992). However, such correspondence or agreement is not that easy to establish. Indeed, some would say it is not achievable at all. We are constrained by the language we use, our limited knowledge and relationships of power. Pessimists, as Simon Blackburn (2005, p.199) would have it, are prone to argue that by interpreting others in our way we impose upon them: 'we annex them, colonize them, trample on their difference, and force them into our mould'. However, it does still seem possible for people, at least to optimists like us, to come to an understanding with others about whether something is true or false – even where there are differences in power. Here the central process is conversation. Hans-Georg Gadamer has described conversation thus:

> [It] is a process of two people understanding each other. Thus it is a characteristic of every true conversation that each opens himself to the other person, truly accepts his point of view as worthy of consideration and gets inside the other to such an extent that he understands not a particular individual, but what he says. The thing that has to be grasped is the objective rightness or otherwise of his opinion, so that they can agree with each other on a subject. (Gadamer 1979, p.347)

In such conversation, knowledge arises out of interaction. In interaction we have to be prepared to question our beliefs and ideas, and be open to thinking about and evaluating the claims others make (see also Habermas 1984; Smith 1994, pp.40–61). Without this there cannot be movement and, hence, understanding and insight. The conversation can take a variety of forms. It can be directly with another, for example, or with what a writer says in a book. Coming from a different position, but still using many of the same ideas, Parker J. Palmer (1998, p.104) is able to describe truth as 'an eternal conversation about things that matter, conducted with passion and discipline'. In other words, it has to be approached sincerely, and in ways that make for accuracy.

It is one thing recognizing that we need to be open to conversation, another to actually be that way with others. As well as helping us to appreciate the importance of conversation, Gadamer also helps us to work with the prejudices (prejudgements) we bring to encounters. He argues that rather than trying to put prejudgements on one side, we need to appreciate how they can assist us in becoming involved in what is being said. They give us starting points. However, we do need to know they are there and put them to the test. We need to continue the conversation. As Palmer (1998, p.104) put it:

> [I]t is not our knowledge of conclusions that keep us in the truth. It is our commitment to the conversation itself, our willingness to put forward our own observations and interpretations for testing by the community and to return the favour to others. To be in the truth, we must know how to observe and reflect and speak and listen, with passion and with discipline, in the circle gathered around a given subject.

In this way we can develop understandings; work at being in truth. However, we have to take care to leave space for the subject to call us – not to impose inappropriate meanings upon it.

Developing the capacity to reflect

Underpinning much of the discussion here is our capacity to reflect on situations and to develop insights and images to inform our responses. Good judgement requires a developed ability to reflect – to relive and rerender (Bolton 2005, p.9) – in particular ways. Such reflective thought, as John Dewey (1933, p.118) once put it, entails the 'active, persistent, and careful consideration of any belief or supposed form of knowledge in the light of the grounds that support it and the further conclusions to which it tends'. This process does not just mean thinking about particular ideas, it also involves entertaining and returning to experiences and attending to our feelings and emotions. For Boud, Keogh and Walker (1985, p.19) reflection is an activity in which people 'recapture their experience, think about it, mull it over and evaluate it'. It is a capacity that we can work at and develop (see, for example, Moon 1999; Taylor 2006). We can learn good habits and deepen our commitment to reflection. We can take what we learn in one situation to another. It can become a way of life.

Sometimes we have to respond quickly, to 'reflect-in-action' as Donald Schön (1983) described it. Just how 'active, persistent, and careful' we can be when thinking on our feet is a matter for some debate. However, it does seem possible for people to think in time to act in different situations. As we listen or observe another, for example, we may well 'experience surprise, puzzlement, or confusion' in a situation which we finds uncertain or unique (Schön 1983, p.68). We can consider what is happening, and approach some prior understandings that may not have been fully recognized. As a result we can act; we can carry out 'an experiment which serves to generate both a new understanding of the phenomenon and a change in the situation'. At other times we have more time to think about things after the event (to 'reflect-on-action').

If we think about the example of the wise woman with which we began, then it is pretty clear that her ability to reflect as she listens and talks is one of the reasons why she was able to be with children in the way she was. She was thinking about what was being said and left unsaid. This giving of respect to the thoughts, feelings and words of others both meant they experienced being valued, and gave space to entertaining and exploring concerns. What is more, much of the knowledge this woman carried into encounters was likely to have been developed through sustained reflection. It is something that is lived rather than simply gained through transmission. Her accumulated experience of different situations, the feelings and thoughts they invoked in her, and the understandings and ideas she has worked at provide her with considerable resources – what Donald Schön called a repertoire. We build up a collection of images, ideas, examples and actions that we can draw upon. We can make sense of new situations by seeing it as something that is already part of our repertoire. Schön (1983, p.138) described this process as follows:

> To see *this* site as *that* one is not to subsume the first under a familiar category or rule. It is, rather, to see the unfamiliar, unique situation as both similar to and different from the familiar one, without at first being able to say similar or different with respect to what. The familiar situation functions as a precedent, or a metaphor, or…an exemplar for the unfamiliar one.

In this way when we hear, for example, what a child says about their family, we can make some sense of the situation by using prior examples and images. We can respond without having a full understanding and try to avoid major problems by 'testing the water'. We are influenced by, and use, what has gone before, what might come, our repertoire, and our sense of what might make for the good.

Being knowledgeable

In some ways what Donald Schön referred to as a repertoire is another way of describing the state of being knowledgeable. To think about what might be involved in this we find it helpful to return to Aristotle. He talked about three different disciplines: the theoretical, productive and practical. The first is concerned with the pursuit of truth through contemplation; the second with making things – *poietike* – and is dependent on the skill of the practitioner; and the last – what might be called the 'practical sciences' – with making judgements. The form of reasoning associated with the practical sciences is *praxis* or informed and committed action. As Hannah Arendt (1959) among others pointed out, in many societies significant dangers have been associated with putting these in a hierarchy (with the theoretical at the top). In thinking about the cultivation of wisdom it is important to hold each in tension with the others.

When we reflected on what we have heard people talk about with regard to wisdom, three areas of knowledge appeared to be significant beyond that already discussed with regard to knowing what living good lives might entail. Perhaps most obviously – and here we return to our exploration in the previous chapter – helpers have to know themselves. If we do not have some understanding of what makes us tick, it is difficult to see how we can make sense of what we are glimpsing and experiencing in others, and the subjects we are exploring. In our experience those generally perceived to be wise are seen to be in touch with who they are and the ground upon which they stand.

A second area we have observed being associated with wisdom is 'knowing about people'. Those generally seen to be wise appear to have an appreciation both of the human condition and of human frailty (or human nature). The latter entails having some understanding of, and compassion for, people's daily struggles in respect of their own behaviour and how this impacts on others. The former involves insight into the total experience of being human. We are born, we die. In between, we live, are part of the world, and make our lives among other humans. 'We are all the same, that is human', as Hannah Arendt (1959, p.10) put it, 'in a such a way that nobody is ever the same as anyone else who ever lived, lives or will live.' To the conditions under which life is given to us, and partly out of them, to rephrase Arendt (p.11), we also create our own. Everything we come in contact with turns immediately into a condition of our existence. Inevitably, perhaps, an awareness of this, the plurality involved, and of our limited time on earth leads many of us to consider our relationship with the eternal and God, or at least our place among others in the world. A continuing familiarity with such questions and the sorts of issues they raise and a certain worldliness is for many, we suspect, a mark of wisdom.

To knowing about ourselves and about people, we can add a third area, the rules and institutions within or besides which we live our lives. Those labelled as wise often seem to us to have spent time reflecting on and thinking about the systems with which people have to engage and of which they are a part. They know something about the ways that families and friendship groups work, for example. They have an appreciation of the sorts of issues that can arise at work, or when trying to access and be served by remote systems such as health services. In other words, they know something of how things work in society. Some of this knowledge may have been gained directly through their own experiences of institutions and systems; however, much will have come about through listening to the stories of others.

Before leaving this area it is worth underlining just how much we may well know without knowing it – and the role of feelings and commitments. As Michael Polanyi (1958) argued, creative acts (especially acts of discovery) are shot through or charged with strong personal feelings and commitments (hence the title of his most famous work – *Personal Knowledge*). He believed that the informed guesses, hunches and imaginings that are part of exploratory acts are motivated by what he describes as 'passions'. They might well be aimed at discovering 'truth', but they are not necessarily in a form that can be stated in propositional or formal terms. Polanyi (1967, p.4) argued that we should start from the fact that 'we can know more than we can tell'. He termed this pre-logical phase of knowing as 'tacit knowledge'. Tacit knowledge, for him, comprised a range of conceptual and sensory information and images that can be brought to bear in an attempt to make sense of something (Hodgkin 1991). Many bits of tacit knowledge can be brought together to help form a new model or theory (Mitchell 2006).

Being discerning

Wisdom, and certainly moral wisdom, entails the capacity to evaluate and judge (Kekes 1995, pp.14–15). Judgement in this context is a process 'by which a decision is reached about what to do or not do' given the good that someone wants to achieve, and their concrete situation (p.26). Evaluation entails putting some value on things. It involves us, according to Elliot W. Eisner, in developing as connoisseurs and critics.

Connoisseurship, as Eisner (1998, p.63) put it, is 'the art of appreciation'. He argues that it can be 'displayed in any realm in which the character, import, or value of objects, situations, and performances is distributed and variable'. The word 'connoisseurship' comes from the Latin *cognoscere*, to know. It involves the ability to see, not merely to look. To do this we have to develop the ability to name and appreciate the different dimensions of situations and experiences, and the way they relate one to another. We have to be able to draw upon, and make use of, a wide array of information. We also have to be able to place our experiences and understandings in a wider context, and connect them with our values and commitments. Connoisseurship is, thus, something that needs to be worked at – but it is not simply a technical exercise.

Those who educate and counsel need, however, to become something more than connoisseurs. They need to become critics. Where connoisseurship is the art of appreciation, 'criticism is the art of disclosure' (Eisner 1985, p.92). It has as its end, as John Dewey (1933) put it, the re-education of perception.

> Thus…connoisseurship provides criticism with its subject matter. Connoisseurship is private, but criticism is public. Connoisseurs simply need to appreciate what they encounter. Critics, however, must render these qualities vivid by the artful use of critical disclosure. (Eisner 1985, p.93)

Criticism can be approached as the process of enabling others to see the qualities of something. As Eisner (1998, p.6) again puts it, 'effective criticism functions as the midwife to perception. It helps it come into being, then later refines it and helps it to become more acute'. The significance of this for those who are called upon to explore questions with others is, thus, clear. They also need to develop the ability to work with both themselves and others so as to discover the truth in situations, experiences and phenomena.

This leads us back to the question of judgement. More particularly, it takes us to the area of practical wisdom. When engaging with what others bring to us we are, effectively, beginning with a question or situation rather than some plan or design. There is 'no routine, rule-governed method, no formalizable technique' (Kekes 1995, p.73) for getting the descriptions right, and dealing with the uncertainties with regard to the knowledge we have. As a result we need judgement. We need to be able to see things clearly; and to make enriching choices. To do the last of these it is necessary to think about the particular situation in the light of our understanding of what is good. In this, as for Aristotle, we believe we should look to be guided by a moral disposition to act truly and rightly; a concern to further human well-being and the good life (what the ancient Greeks called *phronesis*). We also need to have some sense of how our vision of the good matches with others. Is our understanding in line with others in our 'community of practice'? Would other priests or workers come to broadly the same conclusions? How does it chime with members of the groups we are connected with?

This ability to perceive clearly and to make good judgements is what we are here describing as discernment. It involves a certain artistry. For Donald Schön (1987, p.13) such artistry is an exercise of intelligence, a kind of knowing. Through reflection we are able to develop maxims about, for example, working with an individual. We also develop 'habits of the heart' (de Tocqueville 1994) – mores that allow us to function. To this can be added tacit knowledge – conceptual and sensory information that we are barely aware of – and the overt theories that we take from others. Artistry entails the mixing, often not consciously, of these and their expression in action.

One danger in all this is that we attempt to do too much too soon; that we try too hard to understand. Artistry and discernment require both patience and the ability to allow wisdom to emerge. Often when exploring an issue or question we can tread on sensitive ground, frighten people around, for example, the consequences of their behaviour, and ask them to think about things in ways that do not fit with their socialization and the norms of their local networks. While we may 'see' something clearly about their situation, they may well need time and space to approach it. We may also be wrong. Our initial or continuing understanding of their situation can easily miss key dynamics and factors. An orientation that disposes us to wait while people entertain difficult feelings and ideas, and then try to work things out, seems essential if we are to avoid treating others as objects. However, sometimes decisions need to be taken quickly and it might be necessary to bring this to people's attention. Alongside patience we need to avoid working too hard on understanding something. There are a couple of dynamics in play here. First, we can become wrapped up in the detail, the minutiae, of situations and in so doing miss the essential truth. We have to be able to stand back from the situation and see the 'big picture'. Second, as Palmer (1998) and others have stressed, often truth 'emerges'. It becomes present to us. By jumping to a conclusion and not being open to possibility we impose meaning on something rather than allowing the subject to speak to us.

Conclusion

In this chapter we have explored some of the qualities that are associated with being wise. We have suggested that wisdom is usually associated by others with particular people rather than claimed by them. We have also argued that wisdom entails:

- an appreciation of what living a good life might entail

- being open to truth in its various guises and allowing subjects to speak to us

- developing the capacity to reflect

- being knowledgeable, especially about ourselves, around 'what makes people tick' and the systems of which we are a part

- being discerning – able to evaluate and judge situations (to do this we have to develop as connoisseurs and critics).

Our argument is that those of us who are called upon to be helpers should strive to realize, extend and be at home with their talents in all these areas. This does place a particular demand upon us to 'grow with the job' (Milson 1968); to reflect and engage with questions and issues, our own responses to them, and the way others think and feel about them. We return to this theme in Chapter 6. In the meantime we turn to relating to others. After all, people can only be experienced as wise if they are able to be wise with others.

Further reading and web support

- Eisner, E.W. (1998) *The Enlightened Eye: Qualitative Inquiry and the Enhancement of Educational Practice.* Upper Saddle River, NJ: Merrill. This is a helpful exploration of connoisseurship and criticism in the context of research and teaching.

- Haidt, J. (2006) *Happiness Hypothesis: Putting Ancient Wisdom to the Test of Modern Science.* London: Arrow. This is a clear, insightful and inspiring exploration of basic questions around what we should do, how we should live and whom we should be. He shows how ideas around virtue and morality have narrowed, and why ancient ideas may hold promise.

- Schön, D. (1983) *The Reflective Practitioner: How Professionals Think in Action.* London: Temple Smith. This is an influential and very well-written book that still repays reading. Schön examines the nature of professional knowledge, professional contexts and reflection-in-action. He looks at the move from technical rationality to reflection-in-action. However, one of the standout features of the book is his entertaining use of case studies to explore professional judgement.

Further material on the themes in this chapter can be found on our web support page: www.infed.org/helping/being_wise.htm

4 Relating to Others

Relationship is central to the activities of the helpers that are our focus. Many are part of a web of relationships in a particular community or setting. They might well know some members of the families of the people that approach them for help, or some friends and associates. They may also be experienced by a person in a number of roles. For example, Heather worked for a time as a support worker within a housing project. At one point she might be listening to someone trying to make sense of their drug habit; at another trying to encourage them to pay their rent; and at yet another sharing a meal with them and talking about the latest events on a reality show. Handling this mix and the movement between roles requires some sophistication and is often uncomfortable. However, the struggle to make sense of relationships within such a setting holds considerable possibility.

Relationship is also significant both as an aim – *learning for relationship,* and a means – *learning through relationship.* Many of those we talked to in the course of writing this book saw the ability to develop good and satisfying relationships (with our selves, others, the world and the transcendental) as a fundamental reason for fostering learning. By working to improve the quality of people's relationships it could be argued that we can enhance the hopefulness required to remain curious and open to new experiences, and the capacity to see connections and discover meanings (Salzberger-Wittenberg *et al.* 1983, p.ix). Relationships are a basic source of learning. When we pay attention to them, we can both respond in better ways and open up new avenues.

In this chapter we want to explore 'relationship', and what is special about the relationships that helpers form. We suggest at their core are connection and space. Connection flows from shared focus, mutuality and the emotional bond between people; space allows truth to speak, be heard, and be acted upon.

Relationship for starters

Relationship is one of those words often used, but taken for granted. We 'know' what it means. We know relationships are important. We know relationships can be difficult. We know relationships can bring great happiness and sadness. But what actually is a relationship in the context of human behaviour?

George Goetschius and Joan Tash (1967, p.137), in one of the great texts of British youth work, provide us with a good starting point. They define a relationship as 'a connection between two people in which some sort of exchange takes place'. In other words, there is a link between people and it involves interaction. That connection may be something that we are born into, such as is the case with families. It might also arise out of a particular need. A classic example here is in the marketplace. We might want to buy bread, so we look for someone who can sell us it. The two sides have different interests (buying and selling) but they can come together as their interests are compatible. There is advantage to both in the link. The nature of the exchange is also clear – bread for money.

At this sort of level there is very little emotion involved. As Goetschius and Tash (1967, p.137) said, a relationship 'may be verbal, emotional, physical or intellectual, and is often all of these'. They further commented:

> It may include an exchange of ideas, skills, attitudes or values, or even the exchange of things – money, tools or food. Relationships 'happen' at all times, in all places, in all parts of society, and in all phases of the development of individuals. We are involved in relationships all the time.

Yet while relationships are an everyday experience, even apparently simple ones such as buying and selling are complex as they entail cooperation and trust.

We have to work to deepen cooperation and establish trust (see, for example, Duck 1999). By acting consistently and with integrity, often over a period of time, others come to see us as reliable. For example, as workers in a neighbourhood, our reputation grows as we become known for turning up when we say we would, respecting confidences and being ready to put ourselves out for people. If we work at ensuring that our interactions with others are clear, accommodating, and marked by a concern with their feelings and interests, then cooperation is more likely to flourish. Fortunately, we are generally helped in this by our social instincts. As Robert Lane (2000, p.83) has argued, people are 'made for companionship and group living'. Affiliation has a significant 'biochemical base'. There is evidence of common genetic inheritances, and of genes that govern bonding behaviour. In this way, people come into the world with 'predispositions to learn how to cooperate, to discriminate the trustworthy from the treacherous, to commit themselves to be trustworthy, to earn good reputations, to exchange goods and information, and to divide labour' (Ridley 1997, p.249). This is significant. Cultivating reciprocity, honesty and trust is less about building alien institutions and structures than about creating the conditions for their emergence. Relationships are strongly influenced by context. As a result we need to pay careful attention to the environments that we help create.

While many of the relationships we have are of a fairly distanced kind (as for example with neighbours in a street or block), others are wrapped up with significant feelings toward another. Thus, Helen Perlman (1979, p.23) talked about relationship as 'a human being's feeling or sense of emotional bonding with another'. She continued:

> It leaps into being like an electric current, or it emerges and develops cautiously when emotion is aroused by and invested in someone or something and that someone or something 'connects back' responsively. We feel 'related' when we feel at one with another (person or object) in some heartfelt way.

This feeling of being 'related' or connected is very significant to us and to many of the helpers we come across. In part this is because such a personal relationship contributes toward well-being. As Anita Vangelisti and Daniel Perlman (2006, p.3) remind us, they have a holistic quality: 'They are more than isolated interactive moments. They are more than highly scripted role-relations.' We feel part of something. However, feelings of connectedness have to be mediated. The sense of being at one with another may be felt in some direct way, but in our experience it is often associated with a shared focus. In conversation there is some sense that we are seeing the same thing or know where we stand in relation to one another. Here we want to explore these two elements. First we look at relationships and happiness, and then turn to the shared space that emerges between people in conversation.

Relationship and happiness

As Vangelisti and Perlman (2006, p.4) have noted, there is a plethora of evidence showing that close relations are 'vital to various indicators of well-being including happiness, mental health, physical health and even longevity'. For example, Robert Putnam (2000) has shown that people live longer, achieve more educationally, and are far less likely to be depressed in communities where there are stronger social networks and more involvement in clubs and groups. In a similar vein, Robert Lane (2000) has revealed strong links between subjective feelings of well-being and companionship (by which he means family solidarity and friendship). We gain happiness through our relationships with other people: 'it is their affection or dislike, their good or bad opinion of us, their acceptance or rejection that most influences our moods' (p.6). To all this we can add what we know of the significance of relationship in the early years of human life – particularly in the home. Arguably the most important early developmental need is for love and security. On it, as Mia Kellmer Pringle suggested in an older, but influential, UK survey (1980), depends the development of the personality – the ability to care and respond to affection. She concluded that a continuous, reliable, loving relationship, first within the family unit, then with a growing number of others, can meet this need. Such relationships can give individuals a sense of worthwhileness and of a coherent personal identity. More recently Nel Noddings (2002, p.284) has argued:

> The best homes provide not only food, shelter, clothing, and protection but also attentive love; that is at least one adult in the home listens to the needs expressed there and responds in a way that maintains caring relations. The way of relating characterized by attentive love is educative. Because it is attentive it sets the stage for children to explore more or less freely, to learn things they really want to learn, and to understand why they must become at least minimally competent in some things they would prefer to avoid. With good-humoured help in this last category, children sometimes adopt inferred needs as their own expressed needs.

All this comes as little surprise given that, as we have already seen, people are by nature social animals. It is clear why educating for and through relationship should be central to public policy and to the activities of families, and groups.

Yet remarkably little attention is given to the nurturing of care and relationship in social and educational policy. For example, in many other countries a far greater emphasis is given in curricula to skilling young people for training and the labour force than to exploring relationships, and to cultivating friendship and association (Wolf 2002). As a result of this kind of neglect, Nel Noddings (2002, pp.292–300) has argued strongly for educating for private as well as public life. This concern has been given an added twist by the work of Robert Lane and others. For example, Lane has shown that while possessing more and earning significantly higher incomes has little impact on happiness, many people consistently choose higher income over companionship. He has argued that people 'are not very good judges of how, even within the private spheres of their own lives, to increase, let along maximize, their happiness' (2000, p.9). Avner Offer (2006) has similarly shown just how bad 'advanced' economies are at creating environments where consistent choices can be made.

The reasons for such poor choice lie in part in the 'economistic' cultures and ideologies that dominate Western societies (see, for example, Fromm 1995, p.67) and by the 'flow of novelty' they produce (Offer 2006). However, to understand why people do not choose paths that lead to their own well-being, Lane argues, we have to go back to the highly individualistic nature of selfhood that is common in those societies. In 'pre-modern' or more traditional societies greater weight was and is put on the whole. Indeed, it is very difficult for people to know who they are and what they are to do without these. It is through membership of social groups that individuals identify themselves and are identified by others. With the break-up of such an order in many Western countries came 'possessive individualism' (Macpherson 1962, p.270). This involved the idea that we naturally 'own' our own person and capacities, and owe nothing to society for them. The result is a much greater emphasis on the pursuit of individual rather than group goals, and a more instrumental view of relationships. The latter are approached more in terms of profit and loss – what they might yield to the individual – rather than as part of living.

Other problems arise when we move in the other direction and over-emphasize the collective. A strong focus on the needs of 'the whole' can lead to significant pain and the denial of flourishing to individuals. In addition, where particular groups or sectors of society are able to make their definitions of what might be in the public interest the ones that count in policy decisions, there is always a strong possibility of the interests of the many being subverted. Collective activity can exclude as well as include.

Relation, irrelation and the space between

If the failure of people in many societies to choose experiences and activities that will make them happy is linked to issues around the way people come to understand themselves, then it is necessary to explore paths that take us beyond the problems of individualism and collectivism. We have to think about our selves in ways that recognize that our identities emerge out of our having to deal with the experiences and problems of life. As Derek Layder (2004, p.88) has commented, many of the issues that arise have to do with a basic dilemma – that between 'separateness' and 'relatedness'. At times we want to be away from others, to have our own 'space'; at others we feel a deep need to be with people. When we feel rejected or outside a particular group we may well crave recognition and acceptance. 'In other situations we might feel that other people expect too much of us, always wanting us to do what the group does, or what they want us to do and we secretly wish that we could have more independence' (p.88).

One of the great explorers of this territory has been Martin Buber. In his best known work, *I and Thou* (1958), he presents us with two funda- mental orientations to the world – relation and irrelation. These alternatives are close to what Erich Fromm (1979) later talked about as 'be- ing' and 'having'. We can choose between taking our place alongside whatever confronts us and addressing it as 'you'; or we 'can hold ourselves apart from it and view it as an object, an "it"' (Vermes 1988, pp.40–1). He names these orientations I–You (Thou) and I–It encounters. When 'man meets man', when one human being turns to another human being as another, the possibility of relation arises (I–You). I–It involves distancing; differences are accentuated, and the uniqueness of 'I' emphasized. Rather than connecting with the other as another, we treat them more like objects. We act upon them. Individuals, according to Buber, will move between I–It and I–You (and back again). The quality of life in a community or society will depend on the balance between I–You and I–It relations. Emphasis on the latter will lead to a rather selfish and individualistic society; an over-accent on the former helps create communities in which complex organization becomes difficult (Kraemer 2003).

Buber looked to the 'space' between people. At the root of his philosophy was the idea that self-perfection is achievable only within relationship with others. He believed that 'all real living is meeting' (Buber 1958, p.25). For him that relationship existed in the form of dialogue. Thus, relation or 'the between' is a result, at the personal level 'of the opening of the person to dialogue' (Avnon 1998, p.149). Significantly, for Buber dialogue involves all kinds of relation: to self, to other(s) and to all forms of created being. This way of viewing our selves – what we are – and our relation to the world can be quite difficult to grasp. This is especially so when the dominant idea of what it means to be an individual is very different. However, it is worth persevering with. It allows us to think about how we can be and work with others so that they may flourish and be happy. Here, we just want to highlight two points.

First, and this is something we will explore at more length later, to appreciate who we are, and what others are saying and meaning, we do not have to keep delving ever deeper 'inside'. Rather we can look to what is happening when we encounter people, objects and events. If we, as helpers, take up this view of selfhood our concern becomes *joining with* another or others in looking at some experience or issue. Our interest is in people in relation – what happens and the feelings involved when they encounter this person or that attitude, for example.

Second, if conversation/dialogue is so fundamental we need to deepen our appreciation of it. Here Martin Buber threw light on what might be involved. He focused on three forms of conversation or dialogue:

> There is genuine dialogue – no matter whether spoken or silent – where each of the participants really has in mind the other or others in their present and particular being and turns to them with the intention of establishing a living mutual relation between himself and them. There is technical dialogue, which is prompted solely by the need of objective understanding. And there is monologue disguised as dialogue, in which

two or more men, meeting in space, speak each with himself in strangely tortuous and circuitous ways and yet imagine they have escaped the torment of being thrown back on their own resources. (Buber 1947, p.19; 2002, p.22)

The meeting involved in genuine dialogue or conversation is rare, and is, in essence, a meeting of souls. It involves being truly with the other person. According to Buber this kind of meeting is not found by seeking, but by grace. We are called to genuine dialogue and conversation, rather than actively searching for it. It appears through concern for the other and develops via our attentiveness and openness to what is going on. If we try too hard, if we tip over into interrogation, then we can easily fall into an I–It interaction where we act upon the other (which cannot be considered as dialogue or conversation). Technical dialogue or conversation is driven by the need to understand something and need not engage the soul. It is a very necessary part of life. We would be exhausted (and would probably not get much done) if we engaged the soul in everything we do. A lot of the time all we need is simple information. Monologue, a distorted form of dialogue or conversation, is common. Words are said, but there is little or no connection.

Relationship and otherness

Dialogue involves 'turning towards the other' (Buber 1947, p.22; 2002, p.25). This happens physically, mentally and emotionally. If we look at someone and address them, we turn to them 'with the body but also with the soul'. We direct our attention to them. In doing this we can recognize that they are not us; they are separate, different and worthy of our respect. At the same time we know we are connected in some way. Dealing with the 'otherness' of the other can present us as helpers with a number of issues. Here we want to explore three:

- where otherness is seen as something dangerous and thus in need of control
- where difference, especially of culture, is such that we feel limited in what we can do
- where dislike of the person makes being and working with them difficult.

Otherness

Within societies particular groups of people will be viewed with considerable suspicion and fear. They may well be seen as a threat to order – economically, politically, socially and sexually – and become scapegoats for various ills (see hooks 2003). Recent groups so labelled within many Western countries have included so-called 'Muslim fundamentalists' and refugees. Classically the phenomenon involves defining a group as a 'problem' and casting them as 'objects rather than subjects, beings that feel yet have the ability to think, and remain incapable of considered behaviour in an active mode' (Gilroy 1987, p.11). It often involves creating a contrast by classifying ourselves 'normal' and the other as strange and unknown (Kearney 2003). In Buber's (1958) terms it entails adopting an I–It orientation. A simple either/or division is made.

The grouping isn't just different, it is opposed. Its members are seen not as people but as the 'Other' – something unsafe and threatening. This phenomenon has frequently surfaced in our experience as helpers. On an almost daily basis we encounter fears of the 'Other' in the people we engage with as helpers – and this experience has resulted in people building substantial traditions of work around combating racism, sexism, religious sectarianism, homophobia and so on. It can also be found, for example, in our reactions to particular groups or individuals. We may be fearful, for example, of their impact upon the groups they join, or their behaviour towards us as helpers. The threat others pose may be real or imagined – it makes little difference at one level. The problem often lies in our reactions. Our anxieties and prejudices lead to us labelling them and seeking to act on them so as to contain their impact. Our perception of them as being 'Other' means we are not able to engage with them as people.

Difference

People differ in many and various ways, but we tend to see only some differences as important. This might be linked to some aspects of their behaviour, how they look or the way they live their lives and the values they hold. While we might not define them as the 'Other', we may well feel uncomfortable around them, as may do others. For example, when new to being around someone with a serious disability we may be anxious both about the physical, and the social and emotional care involved in taking them to the toilet. As helpers we also have to attend to people's feelings and concerns about the 'differentness' of others and the prejudices or worries associated with what they see or seem to experience as a problem. Often issues arise because an individual or group feels that because of something about them – for example, their weight, religious faith or sexuality – they are not at all like their peers, or are being left out of things. Similarly, we may have to respond to the actions and words of those seeking to demean or exclude those labelled as different.

Many of the helpers we talk to experience problems with regard to perceived differences in culture, background and experience. Commonly, people talk about how their feelings of distance – of difficulties around finding common ground and ignorance about people's lives and customs – and how these can inhibit them from engaging with others. However, in our experience two important countervailing forces are often overlooked by helpers. First, if we share part of our lives with others – through either living and/or working in a neighbourhood – then there will be common ground. For example, one of us (Mark) recently lived in a tower block with neighbours from a wide variety of cultures and backgrounds. There was always something to talk about and areas of joint concern – the reliability of the lifts, noise from other floors, car parking – the list here was long. Once one thing is talked about, another follows as we get to know a little more about each other's lives and the issues we face.

Second, an emphasis on conversation and dialogue removes a significant burden from us – we do not have to know about everything. We can ask about things, listen to what people are saying. Moreover, as we have already noted, the simple act of listening to another, giving them time and attention can be beneficial and affirming in itself. Indeed, in the world of counselling and therapy there is a considerable body of evidence that suggests it is less the approach or method adopted by the therapist than the fact that people have space to talk (see, for example, Howe 1993; McCleod 2003).

Dislike

One of the questions we frequently get asked is whether it is possible to work with people that we do not like or whose behaviour we find abhorrent. To deal with the last first – using Buber's distinction between I–You and I–It events, it is easy to see how we might seek to avoid or act on someone who has acted in a way that we find repellent. An example here is child abuse. We may feel that a person we believe to be an abuser doesn't deserve our cooperation in a respectful exploration of their feelings and behaviour. Our priorities lie with the protection of children. It does seem unlikely, at first sight, for us to be able to be in an I–You relationship with such a person. If we need to explore and gain some understanding of what is going on for the abuser we might reason that it is possible to engage in what Buber described as technical dialogue. However, that is still likely to leave us with strong feelings (that also probably spill over in some way into our conversation) and a whole set of questions. One of these may well be whether they have 'got off' on our attention (and our interventions, thus, were simply further episodes in the abuse) or whether they helped in some small way to contain their behaviour.

A more common experience for helpers is their not liking someone that they need to be around and work with. Not enjoying the company of another person generally makes the task of being around them wearing. It is also likely that conversations will be of a more technical or surface kind and will not involve the meeting of souls! The initial challenge for us in these situations is to find things about the person that we can relate to, appreciate or understand. It is also to look to the subject between us. We may need to consider just how much of the dislike experienced actually relates to the person in front of us. In other words, the issue could be that the person in some way reminds us of another situation and this in turn causes us to import feelings and judgements that have little relevance. We may also hope that shared activity and conversations over time will help deepen what Perlman (1979, p.23) described as our feeling for, or sense of emotional bonding with, the other. However, one outcome may well be our recognizing that it is only possible to cover certain ground with the person before negative feelings kick in – and this may well be mutual!

Relating to others as helpers

We have been exploring the idea that a concern for connectivity and space for truth should lie at the heart of the relationships that helpers build. It is a theme echoed by Parker J. Palmer. Educators – and by extension helpers –

he argued should strive to build 'communities of truth'. In those communities, he continued, 'the connective core of all our relationships is the significant subject itself – not intimacy, not civility, not accountability, not the experts, but the power of the living subject' (Palmer 1998, p.103). Hans-Georg Gadamer (1979) made a similar point when he argued that in true conversation it is the conversation that leads participants rather than the other way round. To take our exploration further and, in particular, to help us think about the nature of the connection involved, we have turned to Felix Biestek. His book *The Casework Relationship* – which first appeared fifty years ago (1957) – still provides a useful starting point. In it Biestek argues that while interpersonal relationships have similarities, each has its special features. He suggests a number of questions (Biestek 1961, pp.5–6):

- *What is the purpose of the relationship?* The purpose will largely determine its nature and qualities. For instance, the purpose of parent–child and the caseworker–client relationships immediately suggest many differences.

- *Are both parties on terms of equality, are the benefits resulting from the relationship mutual?* They usually are in a friend–friend relationship but not in the teacher–pupil or leader–follower relationship.

- *Is there an emotional component in the relationship?* It is present in the parent–child relationship but usually absent in the ticket-agent–traveller relationship.

- *Is it a professional relationship, such as physician–patient, or non-professional, as between friend–friend?*

- *What is the normal duration of the relationship?* The teacher–pupil is temporary; friend–friend may be temporary or permanent; the parent–child relationship is lifelong.

If we consider these features with regard to the helpers we are concerned with here (Biestek looked at the traditional casework relationship) then a number of interesting aspects appear. To rephrase Biestek, the helping relationship differs from others on a number of points. It differs from the parent–child relationship in that it is often temporary, and the emotional content is not so deep and penetrating. It has some things in common with what we have come to know as friend–friend relationships in Western societies, but need not have quite the same degree of reciprocity. While there is some mutuality in the exchange – helpers may learn as well as the 'helped' – the fundamental focus of the exchange for helpers should be the learning and development of others.

A further dynamic arises out of the extent to which both parties are active. It could be said, for example, that arguably most doctor–patient relationships are characterized by a fair degree of passivity on the part of the patient. They are the receivers of the doctor's services. Patients have to cooperate, but it is the skills and medicines of the doctor that are seen to do the curing (Biestek 1961, p.6). In a similar way, much schooling takes the form of transmission – the attempt on the part of teachers to pass on their knowledge to their students (what Freire (1972) famously called 'banking' as educators are trying to make 'deposits' in educatees). There are, of course, many who argue against such a submissive model of medicine and schooling. The helpers that we are concerned with would generally expect those who come to them to be active in deepening understanding and fashioning responses. Indeed, we could argue that little is achievable unless they are.

If we go down Biestek's list when considering what these helpers do, then we might reach the following conclusions.

1. The fundamental purpose of the relationship lies in the fostering of learning in others and their capacity to act for the good

There are two important initial elements here as we have seen. First, through the relationships people make they learn about the interests, issues or enthusiasms that have brought them together. For example, a hostel worker may encourage a group to take part in an 'adventure weekend'. As part of that experience the worker may invite them to try canoeing. Because of the relationship they have with the worker, the group is willing to try new activities. The worker may also encourage them to reflect upon the experience and to gain new understandings. Second, a significant part of the learning will be about the experience of relationships themselves. If we take our example further, it is quite likely that the worker will ask people to think about the relationships in the group (if they need any encouragement!) – how they work together and treat each other, who takes leadership roles and so on. In other words, people learn about relationship through being in relationship. The learning involved is oriented to enhancing people's capacity to act for the good; to be happy in themselves and to live their lives so that others may also flourish.

2. There is a strong degree of equality and mutuality involved

The helping relationship should be one where people encounter each other as subjects rather than the helper seeking to act upon the other as an object. This is a point that writers like Martin Buber and Paulo Freire make with some force. However, we cannot get away with the fact that those called upon to teach and counsel have expertise and are generally seen as knowledgeable (see Chapter 3). For many helpers this expertise may well be around an appreciation of the nature of human relationships and human flourishing, the 'ways of the world', and in some specialist areas such as theology, income support or the process of learning. All this is not to deny that our partners in the encounter do not also come with expertise and understanding in particular areas. Indeed, it is important to recognize the encounter as dialogue.

3. There is a significant emotional content

Fundamental emotions are involved in learning and change, and run through the relationships of helpers and helped. Learning and change can be painful as well as exciting. Helpers, thus, have a particular role to play in creating environments in which powerful feelings of fear and pain can be contained. They may well try to create places of sanctuary, spaces where people feel safe. One aspect of this is people having some sense that they are away from the things that cause them pain or concern. Here they need the other people in the setting to treat them with respect, to be tolerant, and to give them room. An important feature of this is for helpers to acknowledge people's pain and difficulties, but not to push and prod unnecessarily. Sanctuary doesn't involve sweeping issues under the carpet, but rather creating the conditions so that people can talk when they are ready. This often involves helpers in treading a fine line between quietness and encouraging conversation. Often powerful feelings are contained because people feel they are with someone who is safe, who will not condemn them for the emotions they are experiencing or the things they have done. One helpful way of thinking about this is as offering a 'holding environment or relationship' that gives people security 'in their vulnerability, crisis or doubt' (Ross 2003, p.11).

This brings us squarely to the person and disposition of the helper. As we have seen, Carl Rogers argued, among the 'core conditions' for a helping or learning relationship to work in meaningful ways, the 'realness' of helpers, their abilities to prize and accept, and capacities to appreciate what people may be feeling, have to be experienced by the other (Rogers 1967, pp.304–11).

A further key aspect of such helping or learning relationships is the extent to which 'transference' may be present. Freud argued that transference lies at the core of the therapeutic relationship – but it also can be a significant part of helping relationships. In therapy it entails patients placing 'the intense feelings associated with parents and other authority figures' onto the therapist (Tennant 1997, pp.23–4).

> We mean a transference of feelings on to the person of the doctor, since we do not believe that the situation in the treatment could justify the development of such feelings. We suspect, upon the contrary, that the whole readiness for these feelings is derived from elsewhere, that they were already present in the patient and, upon the opportunity offered by the analytical treatment, are transferred on to the person of the doctor. (Freud 1973, p.494)

In other words, in a helping relationship – as many of us are painfully aware – all sorts of things might be 'placed upon' helpers. They may come to represent in some way someone else who is significant to the experience of the people they are working with. Exploring how people see us as helpers may well give us some clues about people's other relationships.

4. The relationship is complex and does not sit well within dominant notions of professionalism

Helpers may be specially trained and paid to work with individuals and groups, or they may be helpers by virtue of the relationships they have. Parents, for example, often teach their children, or join with them in 'learning' conversations. This involves them in establishing and maintaining a role as a helper. However, this is often more easily said than achieved. Many of the helpers we are concerned with operate in settings where they have to work very hard at being recognized as people who can be approached for learning and exploration. An agency may well employ them as, say, a key worker within a hostel or day centre. As such they may well be drawing upon an understanding of a role derived from social work or care management – and be seen as people who monitor and manage behaviour rather than helping people to explore and learn. Similar conflicts can arise within youth work, community development and other agencies. There is a further struggle in terms of working with the project member, participant or client. They may well come to the group or the setting not recognizing it as a helping setting. For example, they may have wanted to take part in a particular activity or interest such as a sport or some sort of creative arts. Deepening their abilities in football, say, may well be part of their agenda, but they may not see the worker in the group as someone in whom they confide and explore their situation. What we have here is a classic question of role. The helper is seeking to establish himself or herself in that role – and they need that role to be accepted by others if they are to function. As we know, behaviour directed at helpers may well derive from the way people see and experience their role, rather than the people they are.

Last, and as we have already seen, the sorts of helpers who are around in local communities and institutions often do not fit comfortably within traditional bureaucratic notions of professionalism. Many have a calling. One important element of this is often the capacity to care for people and to befriend them. Furthermore, the setting for their work is often one in which friendship is important. According to Biestek's formulation, their activities (in so far as they are in some part friend–friend) would be defined as non-professional. To some extent this flows from the way in which people's understanding of friendship has narrowed in many Western societies The word 'friend' in English can cover a range of close informal relationships. This means that its use without qualification 'can be highly ambiguous' (Pahl 2000, p.1). In thinking about this we have found it helpful, like Bellah *et al.* (1996, p.115), to return to Aristotle (others such as Mark Vernon (2007) have gone via Socrates and Plato). For him the idea of friendship had three components: 'Friends must enjoy each other's company, they must be useful to one another, and they must share a common commitment to the good.' In contemporary Western societies we tend to define friendship in terms of the first component, and find the notion of utility difficult to place within friendship. It is often seen as particularly problematic within helping relationships. In one classic formulation we can be friendly, but are not a friend. To a significant extent this has arisen as the notion of professionalism in this field has become increasingly domi-nated by bureaucratic concerns, and where more 'helping' takes place within state-sponsored institutions (Smith and Smith 2002).

If we consider the actions and commitments of those that counsel and teach it is clear that the relationship between them and those they help can have utility. Both can learn from the encounter – and there may be benefits and a sense of fulfilment and worth from the relationship. Both may also have a common commitment to the good. This is most clearly seen where they share membership of a social or religious movement, institution or community such as a church. An important, and obvious, point here is that it is often a common or shared task or commitment that confers 'friend-ship'. For example, Quakers have from the start been described as 'Friends', and as Punshon (1984, p.1) has suggested, the basis of the unity they feel with one another 'is not doctrine but an attitude which gave rise to one of their earlier names "Friends of Truth"'. There is a very real sense that those gathered to explore questions and issues in the name of counsel-ling or teaching are similarly 'friends of truth'. What is more, as Vernon (2007, p.167) has argued, 'to truly befriend others is to stare life's uncer-tainties, limits and ambiguities in the face. To seek friendship is to seek wisdom.' It is within this sort of framework that we, as helpers, can talk about offering friendship to those that seek their counsel (Smith and Smith 2002). One way of thinking about this is as 'civic friendship' – which is very different from the dominant notion of friendship as a largely private relationship (Vernon 2007, pp.94–119).

Balancing and combining the various elements of the helping role in such settings alters the nature of friendship entailed, taking it outside Biestek's framework. It also adds to the complexity of the role – and to its appeal to many people. Being able to manage and be these different things to people – and at the same time to be experienced as authentic and to have integrity – marks these helpers out as special in local communities.

5. The relationships are mostly temporary

The relationships that those called upon to be helpers are involved in can be very short – just one encounter. However, in some working situations, such as in a school, parish or project, the relationship may exist over a number of years. Relationships can often last well after the initial situation has dissolved. Examples here include ex-club members who keep in contact with their youth workers; and former residential school students who regularly meet with their 'house-parents'. Relationships are generally not planned as is the case, for example, in normal counselling relationships. They can often arise as a 'spontaneous response to someone needing help' (Culley and Bond 2004, p.6) or can be part of a long associational life (as is the case with religious organizations). In retrospect it might be possible to identify a beginning, middle and end – but the various forms the relationships take can make it very difficult to apply stage models (e.g. Culley and Bond 2004; Egan 2002) – although they can offer useful ways of thinking about situations.

Some issues

The sorts of relationships that we are called upon to form as helpers who are around, and can be there for people, bring a number of issues. In part, these questions flow from our role as facilitators and explorers; in part from our accessibility and visibility in local life. People often expect to be able to talk to the local priest or neighbourhood worker, for example, without having to make appointments long in advance. They do just knock on their door, go up to them in the street and so on. This inevitably means that local helpers have to pay special attention to the way they are seen and how they conduct themselves. They have to establish their role as helpers, act with integrity so as to sustain their moral authority, and continue to be reflective and explorative. As helpers they need to both be part of local networks and ways of life and yet at the same time need to stand outside them (Smith 1994). They need to be both approachable and maintain a certain distance from those they are called to be around and work with. Maintaining this balance is difficult, especially with people who have a strong need for friendship and help. Here we want to focus on four areas that we have experienced as helpers and have often seen in the activities of others.

To start, it is easy to fall into the trap of seeing relationship building as a stage rather than something that is happening all the time when we are around and working with others. This failing is repeated in some training programmes and texts that adopt stage theories to explain the process of working with individuals and groups. 'Relationship building' is often seen as a preliminary to developing group work or helping individuals to entertain, explore and do something about the issues facing them. More sophisticated accounts tend to place relationship building alongside other 'primary functions' such as assessing problems and addressing problems. As Kathryn Geldard and David Geldard (2004, p.80) have argued in the context of counselling, such functions 'do not necessarily occur in sequence, but may overlap or be performed concurrently'. It may well be that people are more likely to approach us for help if they already have a relationship with us that allows them to see us as potential helpers. However, building relationships isn't necessarily some separate task. It is something that happens and can be cultivated as we fulfil other aspects of our role. For example, being involved in a summer play scheme may well bring us into contact with a range of people – young and old. Working or joining in together on some activity allows us to talk and to get to know each other a little better. We also, as a result, become known in and are contactable through the local networks involved.

Second, our commitment to be with, and be there for, people when they are experiencing difficulties or needing help to explore some question does often mean that they can begin to view us with some affection or feel some attachment to us (and we with them). Sharing difficult times with people, for example around the death of someone they love, can mean that an emotional bond develops, as Helen Perlman (1979) has pointed out. A significant element of our time with them should, as a result, look to creating a safe framework within which this can happen. Without being too precious, we need to express in our actions a concern with appropriate boundaries. One obvious aspect of this is to remain in touch with ourselves and our role. If we know where we stand, we can be with another in ways that are experienced as safe and grounded. We can provide a reference point, a firm place in moments of flux. Another aspect is to contain our emotions. If we are all over the place then it is highly unlikely that we will be able to be what is needed. This does not mean that we are some emotionless automaton. That would also be unhelpful and probably experienced as inauthentic. We need to engage with the situation with both our hearts and minds, to show concern but at the same time be thinking about what is happening so that people may entertain their thoughts and feelings and later work on them. At some point we may also have to make explicit statements about our role and position. However, there is some tension around this. In formal counselling relationships, for example, helping is based on 'an explicitly agreed, firm set of boundaries' (Ross 2003, p.30). In contrast in the world of local and informal helping – and in areas such as pastoral care – the helping relationship is such that 'the boundaries of the relationship are typically left unspoken'.

Third, and linked with the above, are issues of dependency. Being a 'safe pair of hands' in times of difficulty and flux can drift into being seen as a more routine or everyday presence in people's lives. The problem comes where the other person as a matter of course seeks out our opinion or help in matters that might properly be their own responsibility. A further issue is where the person wants to be around us at other times, wants to join in aspects of our life that we regard as personal, private or simply not their business. We can expect many in crisis or experiencing significant vulnerability to want to turn to another and, perhaps, not to be able to differentiate clearly about what is theirs and what is the concern of others. It is our job to help them to recognize this when they are able, and to be able to achieve a balance. This is likely to involve our drawing attention to their feelings and behaviour in the relationship with us, and exploring what might be going on.

Last, local helpers classically experience issues around the different roles they occupy within local networks, groups and communities. At one moment they might be the local children's worker, at another a neighbour or a friend, or a member of the same church or religious group. They can see people, and be seen, in very different settings. As we saw in Chapter 1, while there may be different roles associated with these settings, if we are to be true there has to be consistency across them. There is no escaping the judgements others make concerning our authenticity, and the general injunction to live life as well as we can.

Conclusion

In this chapter we have seen how relationship is both a medium through which we work, and a state that we may want to foster. Being in relationship allows us to flourish. It involves an emotional connection with another and can animate us. Helen Perlman argued that what we call 'relationship' is 'a catalyst, an enabling dynamism in the support, nurture, and freeing of people's energies and motivations toward solving problems and using help' (1979, p.2). In making this claim she was guided by two propositions. The first was that 'the emotional bond that unifies two (or more) people around some shared concern is charged with enabling, facilitative powers' (p.2). Her second proposition flowed from the belief that many people are living in 'an increasing anomic and depersonalised world'. She suggested that there can be humanizing value in 'even brief and task-focused encounters between one person and another' (p.3).

The fact that someone is prepared to 'share' our worries and concerns, to be with us when we are working at something, can be very significant. It can reduce the feeling that we are alone and that the tasks we face are so huge. Their pleasure in our achievements or concern for our hurt can motivate us to act. Crucially, their valuing of us as people can help us to discover the worth in ourselves, and the belief that we can change things. Relationships can animate, breathe life into situations. However they are not all that we need.

> It is not at all a substitute for the opportunities and material things people need in order to flourish. But it is an essential accompanying condition, because it is the nourisher and mover of the human being's wish and will to use the resources provided and the powers within himself to fulfil his personal and social well-being. (Perlman 1979, p.11).

We should, thus, not be just concerned with the way in which one individual relates to another. We should also look to the group and the life of the association and community. In other words, our concern with relationship isn't an individual affair. It should link to a concern to work so that all may share in a common life (see also Chapter 7).

Further reading and web support

- Biestek, F.P. (1961) *The Casework Relationship*. London: Unwin University Books. Classic exploration with an opening chapter on the essence of the casework relationship and then a discussion of what Biestek sees as the seven principles of the casework relationship: individualization, purposeful expression of feelings, controlled emotional involvement, acceptance, non-judgemental attitude, client self-determination, confidentiality.

- Rogers, C. (1967) 'The interpersonal relationship in the facilitation of learning', reprinted in H. Kirschenbaum and V. L. Henderson (eds) (1990) *The Carl Rogers Reader*. London: Constable, pp.304–11.

- Vernon, M. (2007) *The Philosophy of Friendship*. London: Palgrave. This is a very readable exploration of friendship as a way of life. It does not shy away from the ambiguities and offers considerable insight.

For further discussion of the ideas developed in this chapter, suggestions for further reading, and links to other sources, go to our support page at: www.infed.org/helping/relating_to_others.htm

5 Working to Make Change Possible

The form of helping we have been exploring flows directly from trying to live life as well as we can; being open, knowledgeable and discerning; a capacity to know and be ourselves; and the ability to develop enriching relationships. It is also often local. We can be available to people in familiar places and frequently in situations as they are unfolding. These qualities allow helpers to engage with others in ways that allow truth to flourish and, we hope, those concerned to move forward. In this chapter we want to explore some aspects of this process:

- building communities of truth

- engaging in helping conversations

- nurturing moments of reflection and connection

- teaching and speaking to the condition of others

- encouraging informed and committed action (*praxis*)

- evaluating what has gone on.

Before we turn to these, however, it is worthwhile reminding ourselves that not only do we have to put ourselves in the role of 'helper' – we also have to be accepted by others in that role. We cannot *help* people unless they accept us as a *helper*. This means that we need to conform in some significant respects to other people's expectations. As helpers we have to behave in a manner that is familiar or makes sense to others. They need to recognize, for example, that we are concerned with fostering reflection, learning and change.

in terms of the process of people trying to appreciate each other's horizons of understanding.

One example of a community of truth is provided by the Quaker concern with clearness and discernment. In this tradition, as Palmer (2000b, p.92) has discussed, people take a personal issue to another person or small group who 'are prohibited from suggesting "fixes" or giving you advice but who…pose honest, open questions to help you discover your inner truth'. He continues:

> The key to this form of community involves holding a paradox – the paradox of having relationships in which we protect each other's aloneness. We must come together in ways that respect the solitude of the soul, that avoid the unconscious violence we do when we try to save each other, that evoke our capacity to hold another life without dishonouring its mystery, never trying to coerce the other into meeting our own needs. (Palmer 2000, pp.92–3)

By striving to be with others in this way we have some chance of working with them in ways that allow them to see things more clearly and to acknowledge difficult feelings and experiences.

If we follow this through, then when working with individuals our concern should be to help build a space where truth can flourish and illuminate the subject we are gathered around. However, this does not happen in isolation. The matters explored in this private setting impact upon other relationships. It is thus necessary to think about how things can be spoken and heard in them, and how they may be enhanced to allow those involved to appreciate truth and flourish. One of the big differences between many of the helpers we are concerned with and many others who work with individuals is that they may also be directly involved in some way with those relationships or be able to impact upon them from another direction.

Engaging in helping conversations

As helpers our work takes place largely through conversation. This presents us with an immediate problem – in conversation everything is changeable; talk can lead anywhere. While we may go into a conversation wanting to explore something, because of the twists and turns that talking together takes, we can easily find ourselves in quite another place. Working through conversation also means it is difficult to sequence exploration in any meaningful way beforehand. We have to wait to see what emerges out of the exchange. As a result, we have to be thinking about our actions and the situations we encounter. We also need to balance meeting competing demands and learn to allow conversation to develop and to engage in such ways that express the values that underpin our work (Jeffs and Smith 2005).[1]

On aims and agendas

In helping conversations we may have some overarching aims. However, it is not possible, if we want true conversation, to have formal objectives beforehand in respect of subjects to be discussed and the outcomes we expect. We can quickly subvert the very basis on which conversation flourishes; we can end up trying to impose our concerns and views on others. This is not to say that we enter conversations with a blank sheet. As helpers we will generally have some sort of agenda – a list of some of the things that we might like to see discussed. We can ask people to join us in this – but agreeing on a topic is a mutual activity. Rather than using a detailed plan or scheme for this we can be guided in our actions by an understanding of our role and certain commitments. These commitments should be related to ideas about what may make for human flourishing (Jeffs and Smith 1990, pp.1–23).

So how do we approach the questions of direction in conversation? We may introduce topics, invite others to participate – but we have to work with them to agree the focus. One reference point may be the sorts of issues and questions we have identified with respect to the people involved. We may know, for example, that a person is going through a bad time after the death of their mother. This may then be an item on our 'agenda'. We may broach the subject, or ask a question about how they are feeling. We test the water. If a response is not forthcoming then we could look for some other topic. We may also try to find a way of indicating to the person that if they want to talk about the subject then we'd be happy to listen. However, in the case of many helping conversations it is others who approach us. They have identified some question or issue for exploration – or have a

---

1   We have explored the process of conversation only briefly here as one of us has written fairly extensively about this elsewhere (Jeffs and Smith 2005, pp.27–41; Smith 1994, pp.40–85).

sense of unease about something that they cannot put their finger on – and think we may be of some use. In these situations we follow their lead in response to our question 'how may I help?' Agenda items generally change as the conversation evolves. These items may also tend to focus on what we do rather than upon changes in the other person. We may seek to introduce ideas around, say, respecting the views of others, into the conversation. We hope that people will pick up on our intervention.

Stories, feelings and identity

When thinking about these sorts of, often 'difficult', conversations we have found the work of Douglas Stone and others at the Harvard Negotiation Project a good reference point (Stone, Patton and Heen 2000, pp.3–20). They argue, based on the analysis of a range of conversations, that each 'difficult conversation' is really three conversations:

- *The 'what happened?' conversation.* Most difficult conversations (and, we could add in here, most helping conversations) involve questions or disagreements about what has happened or what should happen. It entails helpers encouraging people to tell and to explore their stories; examine their intentions; and the contribution of their beliefs, understandings and actions to the situation.

- *The feelings conversation.* Each difficult or helping conversation will generally also entail asking and exploring questions about feelings. This involves helping people to express and describe feelings within a reasonably safe environment; and examining their significance, acknowledging them and framing them.

- *The identity conversation.* 'This is the conversation we each have with ourselves', they write, 'about what this situation means to us.' They continue: 'We conduct an internal debate over whether this means we are competent, incompetent, a good person or bad, worthy of love or unlovable. What impact will it have on our self-image and self-esteem, our future and our well-being.' (Stone *et al.* 2000, p.8)

This framework has the virtue of alerting us to some important dimensions of helping conversations. It provides us with a handy *aide-mémoire* when thinking about where we might be in a helping conversation. These items might also be permanent items on any helping conversation 'agenda'. For helpers, however, there is at least one other conversation going on. It is future-oriented and concerns how people are to live their lives (see below).

Attending and listening, reflecting back and probing

When we turn to the literature of counselling – especially that linked to discussion of skills – then we can see that there are, broadly, three main forms of intervention. Sue Culley and Tim Bond (2004, pp.17–19) describe these as follows:

- *Attending and listening.* In particular they are interested in 'active listening' by which they mean 'listening with purpose and responding in such a way that clients are aware they have both been heard and understood' (pp.17–18).

- *Reflecting.* Here Culley and Bond are concerned with the other person's frame of reference. Reflective skills for them 'capture' what the client is saying and plays it back to them – but in the helper's words. The key skills are, for them, restating, paraphrasing and summarizing.

- *Probing.* It is often necessary to go deeper, to ask more directed or leading questions (leading in the sense that they move the conversation in a particular direction). Culley and Bond (pp.18–19) look to the different forms that questions can take (and how they can help or inhibit exploration), and to the role that making statements can play. Making statements is seen as generally gentler, less intrusive and less controlling than asking questions – although that does depend on the statement! Probing tends to increase worker control over both process and content and as a result should be used with caution (p.18).

We will look briefly at each of these in turn.

In many respects the act of listening to a person's story and showing that we have heard what they have said is one of the most helpful things we can do. While listening necessitates a particular disposition, it also entails a significant amount of work. 'It's not something that "just happens"', comments Gerard Egan (2002, p.75), 'It is an activity. [It] requires work.' It is easy to go through the motions of listening but not be engaged, to half hear and to hear without actually connecting. As a result our listening needs to be infused with care and informed by the wish to bring people's experiences, feelings and understandings out into the open so that both they and we can appreciate their position. We hope that appreciation will also feed into work around what we find. This quality of listening, of being with, is not something that many people develop (Rogers 1980, p.142). Part of the problem is that we have to sift and make judgements about the nature of what we hear as we are listening. We have to reflect-in-action, and develop questions and responses that might help carry exploration forward and help the other. Another aspect might be that we are trying too hard, getting caught by the detail and missing the larger picture. There is a case for 'unfocused listening' – listening that allows images, words and phrases to surface (Casement 1985, p.36). We may sense that these are significant for the person, or that they jar or do not fit. Not surprisingly the understandings we come to should be tentative. We may only have heard part of the story; the social and cultural divide between us might be such that it is difficult to fully appreciate what people are saying about their experiences; and our own values and beliefs may be so strong around some issues (e.g. with regard to abortion or physically harming another) that it is difficult to 'hear' what they are saying.

Reflecting back what the other person has said has two key functions. Done well, it shows them that we have heard, understood and appreciated what they have said. Second, it can carry the process of exploration forward. What they have been feeling or experiencing has been externalized. As such it then takes on a different character, one that allows some possibility of exploration and work. Hearing worries and thinking being fed back invites further response, and the emphasis we, as helpers, may put on different aspects may well highlight points of investigation and discovery. The main processes – restating (repeating words or phrases that appear to have significant meaning or emotional force); paraphrasing (rephrasing that, in the words of Gerard Egan, 'captures the highlights'); and summarizing (longer paraphrases that assemble some of what we understand as the central elements of what has been said – are all relatively short responses. As Egan (2002, p.112) has put it, 'the helping process goes best when I engage the client in a dialogue rather than give speeches or allow the client to ramble. In a dialogue, the helper's responses can be relatively frequent but should be lean and trim'.

Probing takes the form of statements, requests, questions, and words or phrases that reveal our ideas about what it might be important for people to address. Sometimes they may be simple requests for further information about the situation so that we can gain a fuller picture or be more concrete in our exploration. At other times they seek to encourage the person to look again at some aspect or to dig further into their situation. Counselling skills such as these, as Alistair Ross (2003, p.46) has commented, are important and can be developed through reflection and training. However, 'no matter how good a person's skills, they must be matched by relational qualities' – the virtues and dimensions of character that we explored earlier in this book.

Nurturing moments of reflection and connection

As we have already seen, as helpers we need to have an appreciation of what might make for human flourishing. We need to have some idea of what is good (and who we are) so that we can judge our response to situations. We have to think on our feet and work out what might be the right response for this person or that. Part of the problem with this is that we are surrounded, as Parker J. Palmer (2000, p.92) again has put it, by groups and communities 'based on the practice of "setting each other straight" – an ultimately totalitarian practice bound to drive the shy soul into hiding'. We have to take care that we do not impose our ideas of what might make for human flourishing on the other person. Those ideas simply provide us with a reference point for thinking about our explorations with the person. Our task is to work with the other person to create an environment in which truth can emerge and be acted upon. Within this we have to be with the other person in such a way that they have the room and ability to engage in reflective thought (see Chapter 3). We also need to be looking to connection. By this we mean the process of identifying links with other aspects of our experience, and of being in some significant way in 'communion'.

In order for this to happen we, as helpers, will often have to work with people to handle or manage their feelings. Indeed, they may well be engaged in a real struggle, with their emotions spilling over towards others. In these circumstances a major concern is likely to be containment. Strong feelings need acknowledging and managing. This may well involve significant work on the part of the helper. Without this, reflection and exploration will not be possible in any sustained way. The image Patrick Casement (1985, p.133) uses in the context of psychoanalysis is of holding (after Winnicott 1965):

> [W]hat is needed is a form of holding, such as a mother gives to her distressed child. There are various ways in which one adult can offer to another this holding (or containment). And it can be crucial for a patient to be thus held in order to recover, or to discover maybe for the first time, a capacity for managing life and life's difficulties without continued avoidance or suppression.

In many situations working to build an environment in which strong feelings and emotions can be contained is our main concern as helpers. As this is happening, it is hoped that some space is opened up for people to begin to think about what is troubling them or causing pain or distress to others. As helpers we need to be experienced as a 'safe pair of hands'. Part of this may take the form of us making explicit questions or statements. However, a great deal of the impact in this area generally flows from our demeanour and presence as helpers. In a very real sense we have not only to appear to be at home dealing with strong emotions and deeply felt issues, we also have to be at home with them. Inauthenticity around this area can quickly show through.

There are various means we can employ to encourage or create space for moments of reflection and connection. We might encourage someone to take time out to write something down; we might have some activity they can do that might highlight important areas for thought. However, the central experience helpers tend to employ is silence. Silence can be difficult to handle – both for ourselves and for others in the encounter. Our discomfort can sometimes get in the way of space for the other. It is, thus, necessary to find a balance between:

- enabling people
- providing space for them to reflect
- helping them to face their discomfort. (Culley and Bond 2004, p.30).

We need to avoid using silence like a weapon – making things difficult for the other so that they are forced into talking about something. Instead we need to approach it as a gentle invitation to join us in peace. Sometimes people will speak, sometimes it is necessary for us to break the silence – perhaps to talk about something that has occurred to us during the silence; or because the other person is signalling in some way that they would like speech. A classic way forward here is to comment on, or ask about, process – 'how are you feeling now?' and so on.

If we as helpers are comfortable with being quiet then this will usually ease the unease of the other. However, it is not so much the absence of noise that enables connection – especially with the other – but stillness (Punshon 1987, p.7). Stillness is a state of attentiveness: 'It involves an awareness of one's being, not one's doing. That is why it is still. Silence is defined from outside, stillness from within' (p.8).

Teaching and speaking to the condition of others

Teaching – organized moments dedicated to encouraging particular learning – is a fundamental part of the sort of helping we are exploring here. There is a place for the direct giving of information, for example around the operation of the income support system; more sustained exploration of an experience, idea or concept; and nurturing skills. However, many of the helpers we talk to experience some tensions around this. On the one hand there is the fear of talking too much; of focusing on the giving of information, for example, to the extent that they are experienced as didactic. On the other hand, there is the worry that that they are not saying enough. The problem we face here is that the different facets of our role as helpers are fluid and are heavily dependent upon the particular encounter and situation. Teaching in these circumstances is something that emerges out of the encounter with others. Two questions are, thus, of particular relevance to us:

- Is this a situation where the other person appears to have a live question that requires specific information or coaching?

- How likely is it that what I have to say will speak to their condition?

The first of these questions concerns whether a 'teachable moment' has arisen in the encounter (Havinghurst 1972, p.7; Woods and Jeffrey 1996). These openings for organized learning tend to occur when a person has said something or behaved in a way that highlights a possible issue and where we sense some readiness to entertain or explore it. It is possible to open up new avenues of thought by, as Josephine Macalister Brew has said, 'occasionally, very occasionally, giving [conversation] that twist which leads it to your goal' (1943, p.16). The 'twist' may take various forms. It may be the odd word that shifts the focus of the conversation. It could involve a change of gear such as inviting people to participate in a more formal activity or 'interlude'. Much of the power of these moments rests in our ability to react appropriately at that time and in that place; to catch a live issue or question. This leads us to the second question.

Having recognized a teachable moment we have also to check ourselves. What is it that we can offer? Is it something that might, as George Fox (1998) put it, speak to the other person's condition? In other words, might it connect with them and help them to come to a right decision or to answer a question? Here we have to balance the risk of saying something inappropriate or merely irrelevant with the possibility of pertinence. We may have some sense of knowing what is going on for the other and can therefore act more sure-footedly. However, most of the time we are likely to be in the dark. There may be something about the situation that leads us to a cautious response. We may have a feeling, or we may reflect and calculate (or both).

Encouraging informed and committed action

So far we have focused upon fostering understanding and the entertaining, containing and appreciation of emotions and feelings. However, the role of helpers isn't just oriented to understanding and feeling. It is also concerned with action – with how people can act with understanding and sensitivity to improve their lives and those of others. One way of thinking about this is as cultivating informed, committed action. This is not just action based on reflection. It is action that embodies certain qualities.

These include a commitment to human well-being and the search for truth, and respect for others. It is the action of people who are free, who are able to act for themselves… It requires that a person 'makes a wise and prudent practical judgement about how to act in this situation'. (Smith 1994, p.167)

Put another way, we are talking about ways of working with individuals that is oriented to *praxis*. It is a form of working with that is concerned with the deepening of understanding and to acting in the world. It looks to the decisions people make, the way they treat others, the things they do. The process looks to participants acting in ways that reflect thoughtfulness and that are uplifting. This is, we believe, what is involved in being fundamentally concerned with enhancing human flourishing.

A central aspect of working relationships is the extent to which we as helpers are committed to change for ourselves. Are we looking to learn and to be different – and to embrace the possibilities that come our way (or are inherent in situations)? Being around someone who has these qualities can lead people to question their own situation and attitude. It can provide a positive stimulus to action. However, if this quality is too 'in your face' it can also be a major turn-off. The scale of the change required can seem too daunting. For the most part, our enthusiasm and commitment needs to be experienced rather than made a focus of attention. We need to avoid the 'I did it, so why can't you' approach.

There is a further dimension here; as we have already seen, our authority as educators is dependent upon us 'practising what we preach'. If we are heeded it is mainly because people see us as deserving of respect. If we are not, then people will ask why they should listen to us, and even why they should bother to engage in conversation with us. Attention to our own actions is crucial (Jeffs and Smith 2005, pp.96–9). This is a very challenging consideration. It demands a high level of commitment and constant vigilance concerning our own actions and disposition.

Committing to change

Understanding a situation is one thing – discerning what is good, and wanting to do something about it is quite another. For appropriate action to occur there needs to be commitment. However, we also need to ask about that commitment – and whether it is concerned with well-being (for the person and the community as a whole).

To explore some of these questions we found the work of Gerard Egan (2002) helpful. However, we do need to sound a note of caution. This way of thinking does tend to pay particular attention to goal setting (having a clear idea of what people want to achieve), and goal questioning (checking out whether the goal is good). There are some issues around this. In particular, an emphasis on goal setting can sometimes tend to simplify or trivialize. It can also work to hem people in. Furthermore, it is often easy to slip quickly into setting goals without properly exploring people's emotional state and motivations. That said, we are concerned with praxis – informed and committed *action* – and for that to occur in ways that are just and enhancing of well-being we do need to have some clarity about what we want to achieve.

Egan (2002) emphasizes three aspects of the 'commitment process':

- *Helping people to use their imaginations to spell out possibilities for a better future* – asking people what they want and need and discovering some of the possibilities. We can use various approaches to stimulate thinking about what the possibilities may be, for example, brain-storming, writing or acting out possible stories, encouraging questions that open up different futures (Egan 2002, pp.263–73). One way of thinking about this area (particularly the last question) is encouraging people to name their needs and dreams, and to then work at building them into some sort of vision. We might also describe the process as encouraging people to look to new experiences or to explore opportunities.

- *Helping people to choose appropriate, realistic and challenging goals* – asking people to consider what they want, given the possibilities. What are their choices? 'What is good?' One of the first tensions that we need to address is the specificity of the goals that people set. Clearly part of the task is to help people to state what they need and want; but the next step that people like Egan take is to argue that these should be put in very specific ways as outcomes or accomplishments. What is it that you actually want to be able to do? In other words, there is an assumption that having broad aims will not drive behaviour in the same way as clear and specific goals. We can see the place for such goal setting – but there are dangers around getting too deep into this too early. Helpers can fall into the trap of trying to get to goals before people have entertained their feelings and allowed the situation and their experiences speak to them. People need to be able to commit to, and be animated by, goals. Such commitment isn't just the act of promising or putting our trust into something, it also involves drawing upon our values and beliefs.

- *Helping people discover incentives for commitment to their change agenda* – exploring what people are willing to 'pay' for what they want; how this will really help; and what it adds to well-being. Moving from saying that we want some change in our lives into taking concrete steps to make it happen is a significant shift. For change to happen, goals have to be appealing – and owned by the people that have to carry them out. Classically, change in one area sets off events in others – and it is important that we work so that people can make reasonable assessments of these.

There will be competing agendas, as Egan has commented, and some important questions. First, there is the issue of coercion and pressure. To what extent does the person feel 'forced' into an action (by peers, family etc. or crucially, by the educator)? Here there are further questions. Is the pressure real or imagined? How strong is it? To what extent is the person disposed to the agenda anyway? Second, there are 'costs' arising out of the feelings and emotions that are associated with possible changes. Our questioning and conversation may well need to bring these to the surface, to encourage exploration and to include them in any calculations made. Third, virtues such as courage and faith are key aspects of the process. It takes a certain amount of bravery to step outside the norm. Taking such action will also involve hope and a belief that change is possible and will probably come in time. As helpers we therefore need to look at how we can work at situations where these virtues can be fostered.

Planning and making change

As Egan (2002, p.336) points out, planning goes on throughout the process of working with others. 'Little plans' often emerge out of conversations – small things that have to be done to realize what we have talked about. Making a call, getting some information, talking to a friend are examples here. In other words, helping people to develop a response to a situation may well not entail moving into a full 'casework' mode. It is simply part of everyday conversation. However, there are more formal moments when we have to sit down with others to map out actions. Such overt times of organizing – and the plans that arise from them – have significant advantages. They help people who need discipline; keep them from becoming overwhelmed by what has to be done; provide a means of developing better strategies; and allow for a deeper appreciation of what is entailed and the obstacles.

From here we may well be called upon to work with the other person to develop their plans. As helpers we may also want to explore people's experiences, feelings and thoughts around what they are trying to do and offer our support and encouragement.

Evaluating the process of helping

Very little that is worth anything around helping is easily counted (Rogers and Smith 2006). However, it is possible to come to some understandings about what we do as practitioners, and what might be going on for those who call upon us. We can reflect upon encounters and situations in a systematic way, and as a result strengthen our capacity to respond to others appropriately. Such practice evaluation tends to be an integral part of the working process. We may think about things like the nature of the interactions, the focus of the encounter, the aims and strategies of those involved, the impact of setting and context, and any possible or observable outcomes (Jeffs and Smith 2005, pp.90–2). As a result we may be able to form some tentative judgements that help us to act. Judgements have to be provisional as there is so much that we do not, nor cannot, know. Significant outcomes often take time to emerge – and are difficult to attribute.

Unfortunately, much of the current emphasis upon evaluation derives from the need of policymakers and funders to make decisions or to justify expenditure. Such *programme* or *project evaluation* is essentially a management tool. Judgements are made in order to reward the agency or the workers, and/or to provide feedback so that future work can be improved or altered. The former may also be related to some form of payment by results, such as the giving of bonuses for 'successful' activities, the invoking of penalty clauses for those deemed not to have met the objectives, and to decisions about giving further funding. The latter is important and necessary for the development of work (Smith 2006). Apart from there being significant difficulties around the nature of the evidence used and around identifying influences and outcomes (Jeffs and Smith 2005, pp.87–90) there is also a basic orientation issue. Those being evaluated tend to want the work to continue. This inevitably means that there is an inbuilt temptation or tendency to present things in the best light. Sometimes this tips over into lying and serious misrepresentation.

There remains a strong case for more sustained exploration and judging of practice. Rather too much of what passes for evaluation is really monitoring. Such monitoring is mostly designed to feed data into systems rather than to make qualitative changes to the work. If we are to proceed with integrity then it is necessary to deepen our capacity as connoisseurs and critics so that we may form nuanced judgements; and look for ways of presenting what we are doing to policymakers and others so that they may better understand, and commit to, helping. We examine some of the key process and commitments in the next chapter, but at this point it is worth thinking about what sort of indicators might be useful in helping us to form judgements.

In everyday usage an indicator points to something, it is a sign or symptom. The difficulty facing us is working out just what we are seeing might be a sign of. Luckily, in trying to make sense of our work and the sorts of indicators that might be useful, there is some help at hand. We can draw upon wisdom about practice, broader research findings, and our values (Rogers and Smith 2006). Here we want to briefly note two key areas where indicators can be reasonably easily identified.

- *The people we are in contact with and working with.* In general, as helpers in a local neighbourhood or institution we can expect to make and maintain a lot of contacts. We can also often expect to involve smaller numbers of participants in groups and projects, and an even smaller number as 'clients' in intensive work. The numbers we might expect – and the balance between them – will differ from project to project (Jeffs and Smith 2005, pp.116–121). However, through dialogue it does seem possible to come to some agreement about some indicators concerning these. We may also be able to say something about the background of the people we work with, and the sorts of things they come to us about – especially when we review the more intensive work we do.

- *The nature of the opportunities and relationships we offer.* We can expect to be asked questions about the nature and range of opportunities we offer and the relationships we form. Here the various aspects of the helping process discussed in this chapter might be useful points of reference. For example, to what extent do the spaces we create resemble communities of truth; what is the content of the conversations we are engaged in and the processes involved; and so on? Through continued reflection on these we can chart what we are doing, hoping to see patterns emerging. This can both feed into our own processes of working – and the sorts of work we aim to do.

It would be nice if we could also work out some sensible indicators around the impact of what we do on those with whom we work. In the normal course of working with an individual or group we can gather material and data – but it is often difficult to evaluate sensibly. Are we actually seeing a change? Were our conversations and activities significant for the individual or group? Frequently, there is strong – and unwarranted – pressure to demonstrate outcomes with regard to individuals. Often the result of pressures to justify expenditure, it reveals a basic misunderstanding of, or disregard for, the nature of social intervention. One of the fascinating aspects of looking back at much earlier research into these forms of helping is the relative lack of concern with outcomes. For example, gathering evidence around individual change was absent from Goetschius and Tash's (1967) terms of reference for their classic research around detached work. There is a fundamental lesson in this. They were writing and researching at a time when there was some appreciation among workers, managers and policymakers of the centrality of relationship, and the benefits it brought (Smith 2007). It was enough that people were spending time around people who could, in the McNair Report's (Board of Education 1944) words, be 'guides, philosophers and friends' to them. Furthermore, as seasoned practitioners and observers they knew that it was very difficult to make defensible claims about significant change in others. Even if they could evidence something had happened – and that it had longevity and transferability – it was near impossible to isolate contributing factors.

The appropriate and honest way of thinking about outcomes is to make linkages between our activities as helpers and the general research literature. As we saw in the last chapter, we now have a considerable amount of evidence with regard to the significance of, for example, relationships in people's lives generally (Vangelisti and Perlman 2006); the impact of longer term support and helping relationships on young people (Hirsch 2005); and the impact of some specific forms of therapy (most especially with regard to cognitive therapy – see Egan (2006) for a general overview). Using such research can help us to make judgements about our practice – and may work with funders where there is some freedom in the way that we can report on our work.

Conclusion

In this chapter we have explored some key aspects of the process of helping:

- building communities of truth
- engaging in helping conversations
- nurturing moments of reflection and connection
- teaching and speaking to the condition of others
- encouraging informed and committed action (*praxis*)
- evaluating what has gone on.

These elements highlight some contrasts with more traditional, individualized models of helping, especially those associated with counselling. The processes we are exploring here can be thought about in relation to working with both individuals and groups. While interactions in groups classically involve dimensions that are different from those found between two individuals, the central concern with conversation, the commitment to certain values, and the basic orientation remain the same. Furthermore, as we have seen, these helpers tend to be located within particular networks and communities, and attend to their functioning. They also embrace teaching, and will often give direct assistance outside of the private space of the helping conversation. In some key respects this mix has parallels with older traditions of social work that embraced casework, community organization and group work; and was located in local, and often religious, organization (see, for example, Reid 1981). However, unlike those traditions these forms remain largely informal and open, and based in calling and often in civil society and associational life. There have been fewer internal pressures in such local organizations and institutions to professionalize and to reach an accommodation with the state – especially when compared with larger not-for-profit organizations (Prochaska 2006).

Further reading and web support

- Palmer, P.J. (1998) *The Courage to Teach: Exploring the Inner Landscape of a Teacher's Life.* San Francisco, CA: Jossey-Bass. Palmer is very helpful in thinking about knowing and learning in community.

- Egan, G. (2006) *The Skilled Helper: A Problem-management and Opportunity Development Approach to Helping,* 8th ed. Belmont, CA: Wadsworth. Love him, hate him – but you certainly can't ignore him. Egan's treatment of what he sees as the key stages of helping is a treasure trove of material.

- Stone, D., Patton, B. and Heen, S. (2000) *Difficult Conversations: How to Discuss What Matters Most.* London: Penguin. Born of the work of the Harvard Negotiation Project, this book provides a useful framework for thinking about 'learning conversations'.

For further discussion of the ideas developed in this chapter, suggestions for further reading and links to other sources, go to our support page at: www.infed.org/helping/making_change_possible.htm

6 Deepening Our Practice

When we agree to help others explore or act upon some question or issue, we also accept responsibility to work with them as well as we can under the particular circumstances. Without this our involvement lacks integrity. Half-hearted participation, a lack of respect for the other, or a want of care for learning short-changes those we are called upon to help. They get less then they should reasonably expect.

As we have seen, if we are not in touch with the people we are and are becoming, then it is impossible to truly know others or develop expertise. Thus, in this chapter we want to focus on some key practices and issues that allow us to know ourselves in relation to others and the world. To deepen our practice and to sustain ourselves as helpers, certain things are essential, in our experience:

- Develop and keep faith with certain disciplines and commitments that allow us to listen, deepen understanding, and respond. These include keeping a journal, reading widely and spending time exploring our practice and feelings in a focused way with others.

- Take our place in our community of practice. By this we mean identifying with and joining with other helpers to improve and open up our craft, organize, and be part of civil society.

- Find some sort of balance or harmony in our lives; making sure we look to what makes us flourish. In particular this means keeping equilibrium between work; personal relationships and commitments – especially around family and friends; interests and enthusiasms; involvement in community life; and space for reflection and exploration.

Here we begin by briefly exploring these elements. We then turn to some key disciplines: journaling, reading, talking and organizing.

On disciplines and commitments

To work well we have to develop what de Tocqueville, writing in the first half of the nineteenth century, called 'habits of the heart' (1994, p.287). These are mores – customs and conventions embodying fundamental values – that allow us to connect with each other, the wider community and the world (Bellah *et al.* 1996). In our experience people generally expect helpers to behave in certain ways. These include being:

- *Tolerant.* That is to stay open to others and their ideas and experiences; curious about them; respectful, and willing to listen and learn (Walzer 1997, p.11).

- *Trustworthy.* People need to engage with helpers in the confident expectation that they will act in a consistent, honest and appropriate way.

- *Good at their job.* As Eileen Younghusband argued many years ago, it is reasonable to expect that helpers care, and understand the aims they are pursuing and the methods they employ. In other words, they should be 'a mature person with knowledge, judgement, objectivity, and a sense of values in social affairs' (Younghusband 1947, p.27, quoted by Jeffs 2006).

There are certain habits or everyday disciplines that can help us to be these things. They can call us 'to move beyond surface living into the depths' (Foster 1998, p.1). In this chapter we want to highlight keeping a journal, reading widely, talking in a focused way with others, and organizing with others. Our choice of these disciplines or 'ways of preparing' is based on our experience of what we have seen work. We know of no reliable, comprehensive and sustained research that could help us in making the choice. However, there is a significant literature and some research around the practices themselves.

Some confirmation of the potential of these practices can be gained from the study of spiritual disciplines, as Parker J. Palmer (1993) has shown. He has described such disciplines as 'daily practices by which we can resist…deformations of the self and world, recalling and recovering that image of love which seems hidden or beyond reach' (p.17). Examples of these practices include the study of sacred texts, prayer and contemplation, and the gathered life of religious communities. There are parallels here with the practices we have identified and an important marker – the significance of 'corporate disciplines' (Foster 1998); of participation in the gathered life of the community (which we discuss later).

An encounter with spiritual disciplines also draws our attention to the role of obedience. Those who practise these disciplines do so to open themselves to God so that they may be transformed. In other words, they view spiritual practices as a means of receiving God's grace (Foster 1998). Within this there is an orientation to obedience. After all there is little point in hearing the 'word' if we are not to follow it. However, as Palmer (1993, p.43) has commented, obedience does not mean 'slavish, uncritical adherence'. The word comes from the Latin root *audire* meaning to listen. He continues: 'Obedience requires the discerning ear, the ear that listens for the reality of the situation, a listening that allows the hearer to respond to that reality, whatever it may be.' Such careful listening is both needed for the disciplines we are exploring here and essential to our work as helpers.

Taking our place in a community of practice

The idea that learning and developing skills involves a deepening process of participation in what Jean Lave and Etienne Wenger (1991) have called 'communities of practice' has gained significant ground in recent years (Smith 2003). The basic argument is that communities of practice are everywhere and that we are generally involved in a number of them – whether that is at work, school, home, or in our civic and leisure interests. When undertaking some task we interact with each other and with the world. In the process 'we tune our relations with each other and with the world accordingly. In other words we learn' (Wenger 1999, p.45). He continues:

> Over time, this collective learning results in practices that reflect both the pursuit of our enterprises and the attendant social relations. These practices are thus the property of a kind of community created over time by the sustained pursuit of a shared enterprise. It makes sense, therefore to call these kinds of communities *communities of practice*.

In some groups we are core members, in others we are more at the margins. Furthermore, the characteristics of such communities of practice vary. Some have names, many do not. Some communities of practice are quite formally organized, others are fluid and informal. However, members are brought together by joining in common activities and by 'what they have learned through their mutual engagement in these activities' (Wenger 1998).

According to Wenger (1998), a community of practice defines itself along three dimensions:

- *What it is about* – it is a joint enterprise understood and continually renegotiated by its members.

- *How it functions* – it is a mutual engagement that binds members together into a social entity.

- *What capability it has produced* – the shared repertoire of communal resources (routines, sensibilities, artefacts, vocabulary, styles, etc.) that members have developed over time. (see also Wenger 1999, pp.73–84).

A community of practice involves much more than the technical knowledge or skill associated with undertaking some task. Members are involved in a set of relationships over time (Lave and Wenger 1991, p.98) and communities develop around things that matter to people (Wenger 1998). The fact that they are organizing around some particular area of knowledge and activity gives members a sense of joint enterprise and identity. For a community of practice to function it needs to generate and appropriate a shared repertoire of ideas, commitments and memories. It also needs to develop various resources such as tools, documents, routines, vocabulary and symbols that in some way carry the accumulated knowledge of the community. In other words, it involves practice: ways of doing and approaching things that are shared to some significant extent among members.

Our argument here is that as helpers we need, first, to reflect upon the communities of practice to which we belong – and ask whether they are right for us or at least have possibilities. In particular we need to think about relations of power and conflict within them, and the extent to which their discourses disadvantage some people, particularly those with whom we work (see the various contributions to Barton and Tusting 2005).

Second, we should look out for communities that may allow us to grow and flourish in our calling. There are several reasons why it is beneficial to engage in this as a conscious task. The process of thinking about the communities of practice around us can help us to name and understand ourselves. We come to appreciate, for example, what it means to describe ourselves as a guide, teacher or friend. We have language about what we do that others in the community (and beyond) can understand. Furthermore, by being together with others of similar mind, we can gain some reassurance and support. We are not alone in what we think, believe and do. In addition, the dialogue and shared undertakings within such communities can enhance our learning and deepen our practice. Last, and not least, such communities can often offer pivotal reference points for judging our practice and the situations we face; and, crucially, help us to keep on the 'straight and narrow'.

We also want to make a further argument – helpers should identify with, and be members of, communities of practice that are a visible and real presence in civil society. This either means developing new forms of 'professional' groupings or participating in the movements, associations and groups where a significant part of community and political life is nurtured and experienced. Communities of practice need to be part of the public sphere (Edwards 2004). There are several reasons for this. First, it is through such networks that they become known and their expertise recognized (Smith 1994). For many of the helpers that are our focus, this is something that is already happening. Their place in local communities is wrapped up with their role in, or connection with, religious and social movements. Second, it is of fundamental importance that people who are called upon to teach and counsel have an identity and orientation that is not tied to the demands of either the state or the market. Their primary orientation should be to dialogue and the flourishing of all – and neither the state, nor profit-taking organizations, have a good record here. As de Tocqueville argued, involvement in associational life and civil society allows individuals to move beyond simple self-interest into the sort of enlightened self-interest that allows for reciprocity (Putnam 2000; see also Sawyer 2005 and Bellah et al. 1996). 'The principle of self-interest', de Tocqueville commented, 'rightly understood produces no great acts of self-sacrifice, but it suggests daily small acts of self-denial' (1994, p.527). Third, and crucially, debates around the sorts of situations and encounters that the helpers face that are our focus are more likely to make sense when appealing to core values within religious and social movements. This means there is, at least, the possibility of some discussion of what might be right and true rather than correct or expedient. In other words, there is a chance that the community of practice could also be a community of truth (see Chapter 5). There are, of course, various forces within such institutions and movements that work against this, but at least there is a set of opportunities for debate that do not appear within the increasingly procedural and outcome focus of state services and the concern for financial return within profit-taking organizations.

Before leaving this area it is necessary to note the impact membership of social or religious movement has upon helpers' relationships with those helped. If those helped are also members of the same movement, religious organization or group then, while there may be issues around power and authority, for example, when a parish member talks to a priest, there is also the possibility of a different dialogue because both are 'insiders'. Where helpers and helped come from contrasting, and perhaps opposed, social and religious movements and traditions we have a different set of issues. There may be significant cultural barriers that have to be surmounted if work is to occur (see Chapter 3).

Finding balance

In recent years there has been growing talk of achieving a 'work–life' balance. It is an odd phrase carrying, as it does, the notion that work is somehow outside life. However, interest in the concept is symptomatic of a reappraisal, for some at least, of the role and impact of work on the lives of individuals and families. More generally a telling critique of the focus on consumption and affluence in many 'advanced' economies has also gained momentum (see, for example, James 2007). This critique speaks directly to us as helpers. It both addresses the way in which we should live our lives and what we can do to add to the happiness of others. Avner Offer, for example, argues strongly for the significance of self-knowledge and the regard of others.

Achieving well-being depends primarily on how (and how well) we understand ourselves. Well-being is more than having more. It is a balance between our own needs, and those of others, on whose goodwill and approbation our own well-being depends. (Offer 2006, p.372)

This emphasis upon self-knowledge and relationship highlights the need to work for some sort of equilibrium, we believe, around five areas of our lives. They are: work; our close relationships and commitments – especially in respect of family and friends; our participation in community and civic life; the space we are able to make for interests and enthusiasms; and contemplation, reflection and the development of discernment.

Our identification of these five areas has been based largely on what might be called 'practice wisdom'. In other words, the framework was born of observation, reflection and discussion with practitioners and others. However, it is now possible to appeal to a substantial research base composed of large-scale studies. We know, for example, of the primary significance of close personal relationships in terms of people's subjective feelings of happiness (reviewed in Lane 2000); the positive impact on health, educational achievement and more general well-being of involvement in community organizations, groups and networks (Putnam 2000); the importance of work and making a contribution to wider society for happiness (Layard 2005, p.67); and the fundamental role that self-knowledge plays (Offer 2006).

Gaining a balance between these areas is not easy. There are competing and uneven pressures – and the temptation is to respond to those who shout the loudest, or require things by particular deadlines. A common result is that either our time for contemplation and reflection gets lost or we do not give the time and the energy to close relationships that we should and that they need. Sometimes both get neglected. In these circumstances we need to hold on to the importance of balance and build ways of working that assist us in that. It also helps to have employers and funders who recognize that the long-term quality of work is dependent upon giving these various elements their proper place. For some time one of us (Mark) has been involved in an initiative working with local voluntary organizations and aimed at developing youth work and cultivating the sorts of helpers we have been exploring here (see, for example, Rogers 2003). Within the Initiative there has been a strong emphasis by representatives of the funding Foundation (The Rank Foundation) upon retaining a healthy balance between family and communal life, work, and study and personal development. It is interesting to examine their rationale for this as it is compelling in terms of the arguments put forward in this book.

There are four key elements. First, they have held the view that if local workers fail to value, and engage with, their private and personal relationships they are likely to be unhappy – and this feeds through into their work and impairs their ability to help others. Second, there has been a strong appreciation, as we also saw in Chapter 2, that local workers and helpers have to be experienced as authentic and as having integrity. If they are not living life as well as they can then the worth of their words, and the way they are with people, will be compromised. For example, as people known as helpers in a particular neighbourhood they can quickly forfeit their chance to say anything meaningful about family life if they are known to neglect the needs of their families by spending too much time at, and energy on, work. Third, the Initiative has had a long-standing emphasis upon 'investing in people' so that they can deepen their self-knowledge and ability to work with, in this case, young people. Training and personal development has, as a result, been accorded a high priority. Last, the directors of the Foundation have understood the necessity for workers to have interests and enthusiasms. Such interests and enthusiasms both offer possibilities around which workers and helpers can work with people, and, more generally, highlight the importance of animating experiences.

All this does have some implications for the way in which we think about managing our time. The temptation may be to turn to one of the many self-help books or courses that can assist us in 'getting things done'. Undoubtedly, there are some skills to be learnt and basic habits formed, but the danger is of falling into a very instrumental way of viewing life. Once we recognize and appreciate that these processes are there to help us to do the things that we need to do to create the conditions so that we and others may flourish, then there can be considerable benefits in developing good habits. As David Allen has argued, we need to pay special attention to containing our anxieties and 'clearing our minds' (2001, p.17).

Journaling

The virtues of journal writing and keeping are often extolled by those concerned with creative, professional, personal and spiritual development.

It is clear that many people have got a lot from journaling. This is Jennifer Moon (1999, pp.14–15):

> A journal is a friend that is always there and is always a comfort. In bad moments I write, and usually end up feeling better. It reflects back to me things that I can learn about my world and myself... On a less introverted note, I think that it contributes to my ability to write in general... In addition, I consider that journal writing is closely associated with the extensive counselling and hypnotherapy work that I have been doing over the years. It has been a support and a resource and a means of exploration...

The claims made here are not exceptional. Such sentiments appear in many accounts of journal writing (see, for example, Holly 1989; Klug 2002; Rainer 2004). The case for them seems strong, but it is also easy to understand resistance to writing and keeping journals. We might not see ourselves as the sort of person who writes about our lives and experiences in the way that Jennifer Moon describes. We may even feel such attention to self is a little indulgent. We may not know how to start, or where we can find the time to engage in such writing. It might be that we resist journaling because it is something that others require or expect of us – such as when undertaking a course or working in particular fields. This said, we want to invite people to try (and retry) writing journals. It is a discipline, we believe, that can yield considerable benefits.

Journal writing of this kind has a long history. Explorative diaries were kept by 'ladies of the royal court' in Japan during the tenth century, for example (Rainer 2004, p.5). In addition, journal writing has been a significant feature, for many centuries, of the search for religious and spiritual enlightenment (see, for example, Brinton 1972). However, in the second half of the twentieth century, there was a growing interest in journal writing also as a means of enhancing creativity and deepening the capacities of practitioners (especially within psychotherapy, counselling and some areas of education). Various approaches to writing and keeping journals were championed. These included those emphasizing structured and detailed exploration such as the 'Intensive Journals' explored by Ira Progoff (1975), and the freer and organic forms examined under the heading of 'new diaries' by Tristine Rainer (2004). Rainer (2004, p.2) talks about keeping a 'natural diary' – 'an active purposeful communication with the self'. Those who do this, 'write, sketch, doodle and play with their imaginations.

They record whatever their immediate feelings, thoughts, interests, and intuitions dictate. They write whenever they wish – for pleasure and for self-guidance'.

The possibilities of journal keeping as an aid to the professional development of formal and informal educators and counsellors were recognized by a number of academics and trainers. There was an emphasis on the use of explorative recordings by youth workers in the UK from the 1960s on, in significant part based on their use within psychotherapy (see Goetschius and Tash 1967, for example). Mainstream teacher educators also began to pick up on the potential of personal-professional journal writing (see Holly 1989 in particular). In part this grew from the influence of the work of Donald Schön (1983) and others around the notion of reflective practice (see Johns 2004 for a more recent treatment). Alongside this journal writing was also an important aspect of the explosion of interest in 'personal growth', and even became a substantial part of the Oprah website in the United States. By the end of the century there was a significant 'journaling industry' with a range of books, websites, training programmes and retreats, and even specialist software.

It is worth reviewing the case for journaling (Smith 1999, 2006). Aside from the obvious use to remember something later, the writing of journals – the act of putting pen to paper (or finger to keyboard) – engages our brains. To write we have to think. Mary Louise Holly argues that when we 'capture our stories while the action is fresh', we are often provoked to wonder 'Why do I do this?' or 'Why did this happen?' (1989, p.xi). However, it isn't just that writing a journal stimulates thought; it allows us to look at ourselves, our feelings, and our actions in a different way. It is a method of inquiry – a way of finding out about ourselves and our subjects and topics (Richardson 2000, p.345). By writing things down in a journal the words are now 'outside' of us. They are there in black and white on the paper or on the screen. We can almost come to look at them as strangers – 'Did I really think that?,' 'How does this fit with that?' In other words, our words may become more concrete – and in this way we can play with them, look at them in another light. Journaling similarly allows us to look at the needs and learning of those we are helping – and can, thus, be particularly helpful when trying to identify who and what we might want to focus our work around. In addition, writing things down in a journal also allows us to 'clear our minds'. Having made a note of something we can put it on one side for consideration or action at a later point. As Mary Louise Holly (1989, p.9) again puts it, 'The journal offers a way to sort out the multitude of demands and interactions and to highlight the most important ones.' Last, and certainly not least, making journal writing part of our routine means that we do actually take time out to reflect on what might be happening in our practice and in our lives generally (Rainer 2004).

One of the charges made against journaling is that it can encourage us to become too self-focused – and consume time in ways that detract from our direct work helping others. There is some truth in this charge (Klug 2002; Moon 1999). Monitoring this, perhaps in supervision, is important. It may also be helpful to share our journals (or parts of them) with others and to reflect on the processes involved. One interesting development in this respect has been the emergence of journaling groups (Klug 2002).

From this we can see that writing and keeping a journal holds the possibility of deepening our self-understanding, and to making added sense of our lives and what we believe. It can also help us to entertain, contain and channel troubling emotions and gain perspective. We may also develop a greater awareness of daily life; become more alive to what is happening to, and around, us in the daily round. At a practical level, writing and keeping a journal can help us with administrative tasks (like reporting what happened, when and why) and with the process of setting goals and managing our time and priorities. The process of writing a journal helps form the sort of habits that are conducive to reflective practice. Getting our feelings, intuitions and observations down 'on paper' helps us to develop us, in Elliot Eisner's (1998) words, as connoisseurs and critics (see Chapter 3). Writing for reflective practice, as Gillie Bolton (2005, p.46) has reminded us, 'is a first order activity, rather than recording what has been thought, it *is* the reflective mode'.

Reading

One of the complaints that we often hear from people who are called upon to educate and counsel, is that they do not have the time or the energy to read 'serious' books and materials. Here we want to explore what reading offers and why helpers need to get into the habit. However, to begin, we should reflect on what we understand as 'reading'. Here, we are not simply concerned with reading books and other written materials. We also 'read' the world; that is 'we absorb, interpret and respond to...classroom lessons, concerts, radio broadcasts, films, in fact all varieties of human experience' (Rose 2002, p.3). It is also easy to fall into the trap of viewing reading as a solitary and deeply individual experience. Much reading is deeply social. A common example here is the way in which parents and carers read with their children. We may also talk about encounters, television programmes, books or articles with friends and colleagues. We may join a book or reading group. As Jenny Hartley (2001, p.1) has commented, 'reading in groups has been around for as long as there has been reading'. However, there does appear to have been a significant growth in recent years in local reading groups with some 50,000 groups in the UK and 500,000 in the United States.

We want to argue that there are three key reasons why those who are called upon to teach and counsel should embrace reading, read widely and discuss their experiences and understandings with others. These are that reading allows us to develop an appreciation of other's experience and situations (what some writers describe as empathy); extend the possibilities of looking beyond the taken-for-granted; and they help us to relax. Furthermore, while we may read the world in various ways, there is something very powerful, we want to suggest, about reading books.

First, let us consider the role of reading in cultivating 'empathy'. As might be gathered from elsewhere in this book we are not that happy with the notion of empathy. We doubt whether we can really stand in another's shoes. However, we do believe that we can develop ways of looking at things that allow us some insight into the experiences and perspective of those we may be called upon to help. One of the interesting things about the continuing popularity of book groups and reading circles is just how central this process is.

> If we look at the particular books which groups like and dislike, together with the reasons they give, a striking consensus emerges. The premium is on empathy, the core reading-group value. This empathy can go three ways: reader-character, author-character, and between all the readers in the room. (Hartley 2001, pp.132–3)

In these groups conversations about books and characters become or merge into conversations about life (2001, p.135).

Second, engaging with other people's theories, thoughts and experiences, particularly when they are systematically or engagingly stated, can considerably enhance the collection of images, ideas, examples and actions – what Donald Schön (1983) described as our repertoire – that we draw upon when making sense of a phenomenon. There is a case to be made here for what might be described as 'great' or 'canonical' literature. It became rather fashionable to dismiss 'great books' – often those identified with the liberal education tradition – in the last quarter of the twentieth century. They were seen as reflecting the concerns and interests of particular, powerful social groups. The focus upon 'great books', it was argued, marginalized the voices of women and those writing from 'non-Western' cultures (discussed by Guillory 1995). That marginalization certainly requires countering. However, as researchers moved beyond textual criticism and looked more closely at how such texts were actually used and experienced by people, a different picture has sometimes emerged. These 'great' books were valued by readers, not particularly for any universal truths they contained, but for the way they allowed them to discover new ways of making sense of the world. In this respect Jonathan Rose's exploration of the experiences of working class self-educators is especially insightful. He found that many of such books were valued because they offered 'novel, distinctive, provocative, even subversive ways of interpreting reality' (Rose 2002, p.8). In short they had the capacity to inspire. It is these qualities that the autodidacts who were the focus of his study were 'struggling to make sense of it all, found in Shakespeare, Bunyan, Defoe, Carlyle, Dickens and Ruskin'. According to Rose, a significant amount of modern, popular fiction lacks this sort of power. Furthermore, much academic and professional writing tends to the technical and the instrumental. A look at the education, social work and counselling shelves of larger bookshops quickly confirms this. There is a preponderance of 'how to do it' texts and rather pedestrian collections of materials around procedures and the implementation of policies. Books that challenge and subvert the ideologies running through such writing are relatively rare. We need to look, as Matthew Arnold wrote in his 1869 Preface to *Culture and Anarchy*, for:

> ...the best which has been thought and said in the world; and through this knowledge, turning a stream of fresh and free thought upon our stock notions and habits, which we now follow staunchly but mechanically, vainly imagining that there is a virtue in following them staunchly which makes up for the mischief of following them mechanically. (1993, p.190)

To this end we need to read widely, to look to writers valued within different cultures and disciplines, and to rediscover and engage with the 'canon' in our own discipline. One of the striking features of contemporary discourses within education, counselling and social work, for example, is the lack of attention given to 'great' writers of the past. Dismissed as outdated or 'old-school', such writers are ignored by many concerned with fashioning the current and new generations of practitioners. For those who want to look beyond the concerns of current 'system-makers and systems' (Arnold 1993, p.76), and who feel uncomfortable with 'stock notions', there are considerable riches to be found.

Last, but not least, reading can help us to relax. We can lose ourselves in the plot and relationships of a novel, and be transported to other worlds. Even the stereotyped formulas of much popular fiction have a role in 'unbending the mind'.

Talking

Here we want to make the case engaging in focused exploration of our practice as helpers with others; to listening to and reflecting upon what our, and others' experiences and feelings tell us. This exploration includes what might be going on for us in our lives that affect how we are as helpers. We want to look at some of the benefits and processes involved. However, before doing that we would like to speak in praise of unfocused talk.

Most, if not all, of us tell stories about our experiences of helping to colleagues and friends. We may also share feelings about different situations and individuals with those close to us. These everyday disclosures allow us to get things off our chests; join with others; and may even, in the act of having to say something out loud, help us to understand what we encounter and do. Talking about our work also keeps others informed and involved. Such conversations help to create and maintain communities of practice. However, unfocused talk can only take us so far. There is also a place for more systematic exploration with another. This has been recognized, for example, in the development of various forms of apprenticeship. In ancient China, Africa and Europe (feudal and otherwise) there are numerous examples of people new to a craft or activity having to reveal their work to, and explore it with, masters or mistresses – i.e. those recognized as skilled and wise. This process of being attached to an expert, of 'learning through doing', allowed the novice to gain knowledge, skill and commitment, and to enter into a particular 'community of practice' such as tailoring or midwifery (Lave and Wenger 1991).

The benefits of sitting down with another to explore ourselves and our practice are not confined to apprenticeship. This has been long recognized within many of the groupings concerned with continuing development within helping. Many priests and religious leaders have spiritual directors; and in social work caseworkers had overseers or supervisors (in Latin *super* means 'over', and vidēre, 'to watch, or see') from quite early on. As Petes (1967, p.170) pointed out, traditionally, part of the overseer's job was to ensure that work was done well and to standard. However, overseers were also teachers and innovators. Casework involved new forms of organization and intervention: 'standards were being set, new methods developed'. As thinking and practice became more sophisticated, especially through the work of pioneers such as Mary Richmond (1899, 1917, 1922), and demands for more paid workers grew, so supervision became more of an identified process (Smith 1997, 2005). For example, books on the subject began to appear, for example Jeffrey R. Brackett's *Supervision and Education in Charity* (1904). Supervision also developed as an essential part of psychoanalytical training and continuing development from the 1920s on (alongside practice, teaching and personal analysis). Significantly, much of the supervision here did not emerge out of organizational requirements. It was 'non-managerial' and arose out of the desire to enhance practice. However, it was the demand for 'practitioner supervision' in counselling that was, perhaps, the key factor in the spread of non-managerial or consultant supervision. By the early 1950s, with the 'coming of age' of the profession, there was a substantial growth 'in the proportion of practitioners with significant experience', many of whom valued 'having a fellow practitioner to act in a consultative capacity' (Page and Wosket 1994, p.2).

Three functions are associated with focused exploration such as supervision:

- It can help to promote and maintain good standards of work with regard to the field or community of practice. It can also be used to 'coordinate' practice with agency policies. This can be described as an *administrative* function.

- It can foster reflection, understanding and discernment, and, hence, the ability to respond well to different situations (an *educational* function).

- It can help to maintain and develop harmonious working relationships and *esprit de corps*; and a sense of belonging to something significant (a *supportive* function). (This is based upon Alfred Kadushin's (2002) rendering of Dawson 1926, p.293.)

There is a particular gain involved in supervision that is outside the normal managerial structures of agencies and organizations. As such supervisors do not need to represent the needs of their organizations to supervisees. It allows, potentially, for a freer and more personal exploration, and one that can explore organizational issues without fear of retribution. However, consultant or non-managerial supervisors still have an administrative function. They have a responsibility to the community of practice, and those who come to helpers for assistance, to work for the maintenance of good standards.

As well as sitting down with another individual there are various ways in which helpers can come together to explore their practice in a focused way. Unfortunately, open, grounded and collective exploration of practice does not take place on any substantial scale (Smith 1995). The nearest that many helpers come to it is in the discussion of particular cases, clients or groups. In this context, the focus is often on the issues and questions that arise in relation to, for example, the dynamics of a particular family or group. What helpers are actually thinking and feeling in their day-to-day conversations with individuals and group members – and how this fits with some common purpose – are secondary concerns. There are considerable benefits to collective explorations in terms of developing our identities as helpers, deepening our ability to listen, observe and ask questions and generating frameworks and repertoires for practice (Smith 1995). However, such explorations are not just helpful, they are, in our view, essential. Judgements about what makes for the good, for human flourishing, have to be both individual and shared. If we individually decide what is right without reference to the wishes and views of others then we are succumbing to ways of working which are self-serving, anti-dialogical, and designed to subordinate rather than emancipate (Smith 1995). The cultivation of judgement is dependent upon forms of communal life that facilitate engagement and conversation about what makes for the good (Bernstein 1983, p.225).

Organizing with others

The most obvious way of deepening and sustaining our practice is simply to try new things, to reflect upon what happens, and then to act again informed by that understanding. However, it is easy to see why we might be put off this. Worries about having to 'just do it', to 'take a leap in the dark', and to work things through as they occur, may hold us back. We might lack the right sort of incentive to act differently, or a supportive context in which to reflect. We may also worry about how such experiential learning – 'education that occurs as a direct participation in the events of life' (Houle 1980, p.221) – might change us and what we do. The fact that it allows for the use of concrete, 'here-and-now' experience to test ideas, and of feedback to change practices and theories (Kolb 1984, pp.21–2), means the process has particular power and impact.

Finding or recruiting others to join us in the enterprise can help. We know, for example, that acting with others can have various effects:

- It can assist in the development of self-belief and the capacity to take risks (see, for example, Elsdon 1995, p.47).

- It can enable us to do more. We can undertake more complex projects and pieces of work (Bishop and Hoggett 1986).

- It can facilitate relationships of trust and reciprocity. In other words, organizing with others contributes to the fostering of social capital (Cohen and Prusak 2001).

These are significant benefits – and help to explain the appeal to many of working in teams, or of joining with others undertaking similar work to develop practice. Of course, many teams and groupings do not work together well, and can create negative feelings among their members, but the potential for something better is often there. However, much of the helping we are concerned with in this book is undertaken one-to-one. The helper is chosen because their personal qualities or reputation – rather than their institutional position – speaks to a person's condition. When living and working in a residential school for students with severe emotional and behavioural difficulties, for example, while we may be part of a team, students pick particular members to confide in. How the team functions around that, and the consistency and care with which it works, has an important bearing upon whether the helping relationship flourishes – but in the end much of the work remains fundamentally individual. We are on our own with the person wanting help. However, by working with others we can develop complimentary opportunities and experiences, for example in the organization of group activities or social space. By working with others we can also endeavour to develop the broader environment so that students, in this example, may thrive and learn. We can also look to others for support for ourselves and exploration of practice.

Conclusion

In this chapter we have explored some practices and issues that we believe can help us to know and name ourselves in relation to others and the world and to take informed and committed action. These included:

- developing and keeping faith with certain disciplines: keeping a journal, reading widely and spending time exploring our practice; feelings in a focused way with others; and organizing with others

- taking our place in our community of practice and in civil society

- finding some sort of balance or harmony in our lives.

We have also argued for the need to move beyond the usual confines of our role as defined by organizations within which we have to function. It is to the practicalities of this that we now want to turn.

Further reading and web support

- Holly, M.L. (1989) *Writing to Grow: Keeping a Personal-professional Journal*. Portsmouth, NH: Heinemann. This is one of the few, recommendable explorations of journal writing for professional development.

- Kadushin, A. and Harness, D. (2002) *Supervision in Social Work*, 4th ed. New York, NY: Columbia University Press. This is a revised edition of Kadushin's standard work on supervision.

- Rainer, T. (2004) *The New Diary: How to Use a Journal for Self-guidance and Extended Creativity.* Los Angeles, CA: J. P. Tarcher Inc. Reissued with a new introduction in 2004, this book is rightly regarded as a classic. It provides a good introduction to the writing and keeping of journals and opens up different approaches.

- Wenger, E. (1999) *Communities of Practice: Learning, Meaning and Identity.* Cambridge: Cambridge University Press. Wenger presents extended discussion of the concept of community of practice and how it might be approached within organizational development and education.

For further discussion of the ideas explored in this chapter, suggestions for further reading and links to other sources, go to our support page at: www.infed.org/helping/deepening_practice.htm

7 Getting from Here to There

The art of helping others – of being able to be around, be there and be wise – is complex and does not readily translate into a set of easy steps or tasks. It involves being able to respond with care, understanding and a concern for flourishing to the helping situation we are in. In this chapter we tackle how we get from knowing what these notions might mean and involve, for both ourselves and those around us, to being able to work in more holistic ways in often hostile organizations and settings. Being able to 'practise what we preach' is a battle for us all as helpers – not only internally, but also in terms of how we are seen and received by others, and the dynamics of the systems and structures we work within.

Helping and educating require self-knowledge. As we saw in the last chapter, attending to the 'inner helper' allows us to cultivate a sense of identity and integrity (to rephrase Palmer 1998, p.32). When placed alongside reflection and action around role, and the relationship of private troubles and public issues, we can work toward a more holistic approach. Whether we have been chosen or offered ourselves, taking on the role of 'helper' requires commitment and can become frustrating. In working out how we get 'from here to there' we need to establish constructive, and sometimes coping, strategies that can sustain us. We also need to move beyond narrow professionalized notions of helping and to embrace calling and engage with civil society.

Some problems

Negative press around those who seek help can often have an effect on the people helping them. For those groups within society who are labelled as anti-social or who are pushed into the margins, helping them becomes not just about tending to their needs so that they may flourish, but inevitably involves justifying your reasons for helping, and often explaining the existence of the marginalized groups, to those within mainstream society. This can be explored through Bernard Davies and Alan Gibson's acknowledgement, in their study of social education, of the expectation that society places on the worker (helper) by investing in them the authority of a professional. The expectation is that as educator or helper you are able to 'fix' people. Whereas in reality, it is usually the case that the people being helped can only have their needs met if the authority the worker or helper has is used as little as possible (1967, p.182). Davies and Gibson argue that social education (or in our case helping), particularly if it is person-centred, is about people taking responsibility for their actions whether as an individual or as part of a group. If as helpers we rely solely on the use of our 'authority' to change people's behaviour and choices whilst they are around us, how are they then able to make the right choices when there is no-one of authority around? However, this idea and way of practising needs to be balanced and, thus, becomes even more complex. If as a helper and teacher we do not assert some kind of authority when needed, be it moral or the more traditional discipline-bound, then we may be in danger of colluding with or condoning the behaviour and actions that we are seeking to encourage people to change and develop. To understand this further we can continue with Davies and Gibson who make the point that none of us has 'absolute freedom' and imposing limitations on people's behaviour is understood. If we allow free rein, then in fact as helpers and educators we become an 'unfamiliar experience' in the lives of those we encounter (1967, p.182).

An obvious example of practice to draw upon here is of working with young people, and we will refer back to Heather's work with boys with emotional and behavioural difficulties. By being placed within the special needs school, the boys had already reached a point in their lives where their behaviour had proved so challenging to teachers and others that they were no longer able to be schooled in a mainstream environment. This in itself had already set up issues around authority and required the adults to work in such a way that they didn't need to rely on their status given by the education authority. Rather, the helping and work that took place needed to be through the relationship they had with each boy. This was not always easy and certainly didn't happen all the time. In order to build order in the often chaotic school environment, some control needed to be relinquished back to the boys. By creating a safe environment where the boys could make choices and mistakes, they began to learn about making the right decisions and dealing with the consequences of their choices both good and bad. Although all did not welcome this way of working and being – due to its often chaotic appearance – it was key in the personal and social development of the boys (see, for example, Harvey 2006). The space to make choices allowed each boy to develop his own frame of reference, which could be used outside of the school environment. However, there needed to be a balanced way of working. It was not always appropriate or safe for the boys to make their own decisions and so limitations had to be set by the adults. Yet this was all part of the learning experience for all involved.

It is important here to note that alongside how we work with the theoretical notion of authority we need to be aware of how the physical presentation of it affects those we help. Erving Goffman explores the notion of 'body idiom' in *Behavior in Public Places* (1963). He argues:

> ...when individuals come into one another's immediate presence in circumstances where no spoken communication is called for, they none the less inevitably engage one another in communication of sort, for in all situations, significance is ascribed to certain matters that are not necessarily connected with particular verbal communications. These comprise bodily appearance and personal acts. (1963, p.33)

Whilst we, as helpers, may not verbalize or practise in the role of an authoritarian, not paying attention to little details may end up sending a very different message. For example, in projects and residential settings people often comment on workers who wear their keys visibly. Although it is often practical to attach keys to your belt or wear them around your neck, it sends out a clear message of authority. These keys, no matter how insignificant they may seem to us, serve as a reminder that there is a difference in who is in charge and who isn't, and which can often undermine the helping that is taking place.

To work like this requires a certain amount of bravery and sophistication of thinking, and it is idealistic to say that everyone is able to practise this way. By understanding how we present ourselves and what this means for those around us, significant helping relationships can be forged. The problem, however, does not lie just with us. It is entrenched in the systems within which we work. As helpers who are mindful of how we act and are with other people, our integrity, relationships and role can often be compromised, both consciously and not, by the lack of space for action within the systems we find ourselves. Key factors here have been the rise of managerialism within education and welfare systems; greater central direction; an increasing focus on individuals (rather than communities); and an increased emphasis upon the routine monitoring and surveillance of people in contact with those systems. One of the main consequences has been a decline in the discretion of front-line workers, and an increase in prescribed and routinized activities (Jeffs and Smith 2006). A key aspect of this has been the use of information and communication technologies such as those involved in the various databases and assessment systems that have found their way into social work, children's and youth work and schooling. As Garrett (2005, p.545) has commented with regard to the 'electronic turn' in social work, work is 'increasingly being ordered, devised and structured by academics, policy makers and e-technicians far removed from…day-to-day encounters'. He continues: 'Social work activity is also becoming more Taylorised: broken down into bytes with social workers, aided by less costly "social care assistants", providing "customers" with discrete packages, or "micro-packages", of (purchasable) support and intervention.' The use of service-level agreements, commissioning and the like has also reduced the freedom of voluntary or third sector organizations in receipt of state funding to respond to local needs.

Within social work and educational settings the shift in state-sponsored work in a number of countries toward targeting, achieving predefined outcomes, and a heightened concern with accreditation and 'hard products', has had a fundamental impact. While, at first glance, some of the elements involved can appear attractive, as we dig deeper what we begin to experience are bureaucratically defined target groups, specific curriculum or issue requirements, and number-focused work. What we lose is the generic time we can spend with people, attending to their needs and promoting their flourishing as individuals, and as members of social groups and the wider community. As Barton Hirsch (2005, p.131) found in his study of after-school programmes in the United States, such relationships 'are the heart and soul, the most fundamental strength'. Emphasis upon structured activity can quickly diminish the quality of them. People can feel that 'marching through required activities is more important than getting to know and appreciate them as individuals' (p.135).

Similarly, the changing emphasis in English state-sponsored youth work has led to the diminishing of the importance of mutuality and voluntary participation and the substitution of an outcome-based model for the person-centred processes that characterize youth work (and we argue, helping) (Ord 2004, pp.53–4). This causes a direct conflict in the ideology behind what we as helpers do. Ord argues, as do we, that:

> Both means (or methods of youth work) and ends (outcomes of youth work) cannot be specified until the young people have been engaged with, a relationship built up and their needs identified. It is the process that develops from this that will lead to the outcomes. (2004, p.54)

There has been a parallel shift with regard to volunteering in England. Recommendations made by the Russell Commission – and picked up by government – largely ignored the philanthropic and 'right action' features of volunteering in favour of promoting individual gain for the volunteer. They also argued that funding streams be centralized and control given to the implementing body of the scheme (Smith 2005).

The problem we have here is that if the agencies who set the agenda for the work do not understand or acknowledge the importance of process, mutuality and local assessment of need within helping, how are we able to successfully, and with integrity, develop space for the work that is actually needed, rather than assumed, to take place? In response to our personal calling as helpers, whether we get to put our ideas and notions into practice may very much depend on which organizations we choose to work for or be a part of – and whether they choose to take funding that ties work to inappropriate means and ends. The problems we encounter in both general and individual terms are inextricably linked to our choice of helping situation.

Exploiting the gaps

Whether we like it or not, our work as helpers places us in a highly political environment. Although we may not be in position as individuals to change policy or directly influence government and other significant sources of power, we are able to make decisions in our own lives, to join with others to work for what is just and right, and help those who come to us to do the same. It is important that we do not give up hope or give in to the negativity we may experience as a helper. We need to work consistently towards improving our communities. As we explored in the introduction, helpers are people who stand out as different and special, they are people who others turn to. If helping is done well and the space is achieved, then significant decisions can be made. It is this powerful enabling that brings about lasting change in communities and in individuals' lives.

Helping people to assert their own authority through small yet powerful gestures can generate small changes in any system. Paul Ginsborg uses the work of Michel De Certeau to highlight this point. Ginsborg says that De Certeau:

> ...advocated a constant *deflection* of power, and made reference to a whole number of actions to which he gave suggestive names: murmurings, ruses, joyful discoveries, polymorphic simulations, and systems of operational combination (les combinations d'operations). Potentially, these could all be elements of 'resistance'. (2005, p.77)

Whilst we may not have a direct say in how the government or even our agency makes decisions, what we can do is to have an effect on how policies work once they come into our everyday lives; and alongside this organize with others to bring things onto decision-making agendas – to translate concerns into public issues.

Through deflecting power and seeking alternatives in the 'micro-actions' of our everyday business we can begin to bring about change (Ginsborg 2005, p.77). This can be viewed as a prime reason for not always opting out of state-run agencies and projects. Although we may often feel we can no longer be a part of the ever-formalizing helping arena and look for less centrally driven work, remaining within the system can provide opportunities to bring about small but influential changes. This is a constant question for many helpers. Do we continue to be a part of something that we feel compromised by in order to change the system within, or do we vote with our feet and opt out? De Certeau again picks up these ideas:

> ...tactics were more important than strategy, and tactics meant being on the watch for 'spaces within which to manoeuvre', as well as opportunities that were to be 'seized on the wing.' Politics was to be a form of daily bricolage, the assembling of minute acts of autonomy which would distance the individual from the controls of a 'disciplinary' society. (Ginsborg 2005, p.77)

Remaining part of the formal system may provide more opportunities to bring about change than there would be if we weren't a part of it. Yet we also need to ask ourselves if we are guilty of perpetuating injustice and unhappiness by continuing to facilitate certain governmental and funders' agendas. In order to work with integrity these are questions we need to ask ourselves on a daily basis.

For the moment, within many northern education and welfare systems, there appears to be less space for action, fewer gaps to exploit. Some years ago it was realistic, for example, to argue that there were a number of places where holistic and alternative practice could be found within state-sponsored work. It was even possible to make a reasonable case for the ability of 'radical professionals' to work in ways that were both 'in and against the state' (London Edinburgh Return Group 1980). The use of large-scale data recording systems, the move into commissioning discrete pieces of work, and the more general emphasis upon monitoring and directing state-sponsored work has limited the room for manoeuvre – but some spaces remain, and new opportunities open up. Part of the problem is that the emphasis put on achieving targets and following procedures in many state systems has fed into a culture of caution. Workers or helpers within these systems can easily fall into the trap of adopting a far too limiting interpretation of what is possible. They do not look to push the boundaries, or test the system. Many may well feel bound by curriculum or procedures, and get caught up in what needs to be done or taught. In the process people can easily become a by-product of the process rather than the focus. This is hardly a new phenomenon as one of us (Mark) found when working on a national project around political education in the early 1980s (Smith 1984). However, in our experience, there has been a fundamental shift in orientation on the part of many state-sponsored workers and helpers which has resulted in an urge to continually demonstrate how they meet state objectives rather than attend to people's needs.

The contrast with our experience of projects and initiatives around helping within community and faith groups is strong. On the whole helpers in these settings appear to have far more room to work on their own initiative and to use their discretion. Many of the helpers who we have observed and talked to for this book work for, or are involved in, churches and religious groups, or organizations and associations that receive little state funding. They have, thus, been less susceptible to many of the pressures experienced by their colleagues within state-sponsored work. However, they still have to deal with the dynamics and quirks of their own groups and bodies. Some are under strong pressure to achieve particular results. Others struggle to handle the competing demands of different groups or sections within their organization. Two particular things have worked in the favour of workers and helpers within such organizations in terms of pursuing work that is more holistic, caring and concerned with flourishing. First, these are local associations and organizations. Working and managerial relationships are much more likely to be face-to-face. Things can generally be talked about and explored rather than justified to some distant system; or made sense of within some bureaucratic procedure. Second, many of the groups and bodies involved already have an overt and often central commitment to these concerns. They look to the good and, as such, can entertain the centrality of flourishing, for example, and are more at home with the forms of argument and exploration that are involved. This is not to say that there are not profound differences in interpretation. Some forms of work are very difficult in some religious settings, for example. But there has been vibrancy around work in civil society organizations. Many helpers and workers have found them convivial settings for work that promotes human flourishing. They can provide a space for creativity of time, space and resource.

Acting with integrity

Any exploitation of gaps or the grey areas is not a licence to lie or tell mistruths about what we do and what happens. Instead it is a way of making the best of the constraints within which we have to work.

For further thoughts on this we can once again look to the work of Parker J. Palmer. As a helper or educator, part of the role is to create space where learning and change can take place. It is the helper's responsibility to work so that any formal requirements are met (for example, what the person has said they want to talk about) whilst at the same time creating an environment that allows 'time for the unexpected even as it makes time to acquire the predictable necessary facts' (Palmer 1998, p.133). This in itself puts us in a complex position and because of this it is important to acknowledge that we are able to create conditions that can help people learn and take action – or keep them from changing much at all. Helping, like teaching, 'is the intentional act of creating those conditions' (Palmer 1998, p.6). This lays a great deal of responsibility at our door, something which many choose to ignore in favour of following a curriculum or pre-determined plan. Yet for those of us who embrace the artistry of helping and teaching it becomes a daily challenge of which we must be a part.

We have previously explored the notion of integrity in relation to ideas around knowing and being ourselves. We established that integrity requires us to act in a way that 'adheres to moral principles', and this can be directly put into practice when figuring out how we 'get from here to there'. When working in a way that adheres to moral principles we have a basis for our thinking and action that attends to what is right, rather than being focused on what is correct in terms of policies and procedures. If we are not able to work creatively within the parameters set by our agency, then we either need to get out, or go ahead with what we believe is right and accept the consequences.

Exploiting gaps and being creative demands the agreement of those we work for and those we work with. We cannot simply do what we want. If we as helpers set the limits and context of our own working environments and ways of practising, then there needs to be trust that we will work with integrity and in such a way that is not detrimental to those we seek to help. We should also seek not to unwarrantedly damage the community of practice of which we are a part or the agency we work for. In making decisions about what might be wrong or right we need to take heed of what others think. Our ideas of what might make for flourishing and the good are personal, but they also need to be located in a broader discourse.

Lying

We may well be tempted to intentionally deceive others (lie) about the work we do in order to meet the criteria that allows us to engage with people in the first place. As workers concerned with integrity and authenticity we have to think about compromising our own in order to promote them in others. The problem with this, of course, is that it can easily undermine the basis upon which we work. Our moral authority, being experienced by others as people of integrity, wisdom and an understanding of right and wrong, is damaged. More than this, lying undermines the trust that is necessary if people are to live together in society. As Sissela Bok (1999, p.31) has put it, 'trust in some degree of veracity functions as a *foundation* of relations between human beings; when this trust shatters or wears away, institutions collapse'. In other words, we all benefit from the social practice of truth-telling – and that benefit will only continue if people play their part and act fairly and with reciprocity.

Bok makes the case for adopting a 'principle of veracity' – a presumption against lying. She allows that there may be occasions when lying is morally justified, but cautions 'while excuses abound, justification is hard to come by' (Bok 1999, p.89). As we consider different kinds of lies we must ask, she argues, two key questions (p.105):

1. Are there alternative forms of action that will resolve the difficulty without the use of a lie?

2. What might be the moral reasons brought forward to excuse the lie, and what reasons can be raised as counter-arguments?

As a further test of these, 'we must ask what a public of reasonable persons might say about such lies' (pp.105–6). Most lies will fail this test of justification. Here we want to apply this test to an area where helpers (and their managers) have often found the need to lie.

One of the classic areas of tension that we have found among the groups of helpers we have been studying has been between the conditions placed upon the work by funders (particularly the state) and managers, and the local assessment of need. Because money can often only be gained when addressing some policy target, and because those targets often bear scant regard for what might actually be needed by people within different communities and groupings, workers and managers are often tempted to deceive funders. This may take the form, for example, of misrepresenting the work, 'massaging' outcomes and numbers of participants, or of simply slicing-off funding to do other work. There are often alternative courses of action – but they can be quickly rejected as they appear to involve some discomfort for helpers and their organizations. One is to simply get on with the work that is judged locally to be right and appropriate, report this, and face the consequences. Another is to try to engage the funder in some sort of dialogue to see what room for manoeuvre might exist. Often the first leads to the other. We have seen a number of workers take the former course with some success and, on occasions, a little pain. Three factors seem to work in their favour. First, the systems that they are dealing with are often inefficient and have difficulty handling information that doesn't fit in the normal categories. As a result, their transgressions have often been overlooked or ignored. Second, those 'up the line' have a vested interest in things looking good and in avoiding too much disruption. Third, many of these workers were operating in smaller community or third sector organizations, and were working with the support of their managers/trustees. As a result the issue became inter-organizational rather than concerned with the manager–worker relationship.

When we look to the second of Bok's questions it is rare to find a compelling moral reason for intentionally misleading funders and managers. Rather we can find a range of reasons why it is questionable. These include the undermining of our moral position as helpers, the impact on general mores, and the way it subverts accountability. While there are all sorts of questions around the nature of the accountability of helpers to different groupings (their community of practice, those they help; their employer/sponsor etc.), we do have to recognize that there are those with a significant and legitimate right to be kept informed about the work we do as helpers. We should not, for example, be acting in such a way that undermines democratic process. A further consideration is the extent to which we subvert the possibility of learning about the nature of power relationships, and of state and other funders' intentions when misrepresenting work. Rather than allowing people to see the reality of the conditions laid upon the work we can do as helpers and educators, we often keep them hidden. Revealing them then entails laying bare our own duplicity. This said there are some rare, but significant, instances where morally we can take the decision to lie. These include situations where significant, unjust and unwarrantable harm may result to individuals from our act of reporting. However, to retain any moral authority in these situations we also have to be prepared to accept the consequences if we are found out.

Questions such as these highlight, again, the importance of joining a community of practice (see Chapter 6) and of attending to what different groups and communities might consider 'reasonable'. Sissela Bok (1999, p.97) has argued that more than consultation 'with chosen peers is necessary whenever crucial interests are…at stake'. We need to be able to undertake our own 'thought-experiments' and to ask the right questions of ourselves; to consult our community of practice, friends etc.; and to listen to what people of 'all allegiances' think and feel. For obvious reasons all this is not possible in a lot of situations. We have to think on our feet, or take time to fall back on our own imagination. As Robert Fullinwinder (2007) has put it, 'You don't lie unless you can imagine how other reasonable people, in different roles and circumstances, would endorse your lie if they knew about it.'

Developing and nurturing relationships in our agencies

In order to create and sustain space for more open, creative and holistic helping it is necessary to spend time enabling others within our agencies to appreciate and understand these ways of working. In particular we want to focus on working with support staff and managers.

Often, as helpers, we cannot fulfil the potential of our role without the help of administrative and support staff. It is these people who will enable us to concentrate on 'helping' rather than spend our days completing the wealth of paperwork that accompanies the bureaucratization of the helping role. Even as you read this we are sure at least one person springs to mind! Yet often we hear stories of workers who do not say thank you, or appreciate that even when the admin staff are busy they somehow manage to find the information we need or help us complete the reports that are due in. As helpers, positive relationships with support staff are fundamental to our own well-being and that of the projects we work in. This brings to the forefront a common problem – if we are to promote human flourishing then this needs to be across all our actions and encounters, not reserved for those who are deemed as 'in need'. This takes us back to the notion of authenticity explored in Chapter 2. If we are to be experienced as authentic by those we seek to help, then we must be experienced in all aspects of our life as such. Being mindful of how we treat people generally can go some way to ensuring that support and administrative staff are treated well, but a positive working relationship requires more than that. Just as they support us in what we do, we need to support them. For example, there are administration deadlines in any agency, reports may need to be completed or attendance figures noted, and it is essential that we provide the information by the time it is required. If we are encouraging those we help to recognize their responsibilities and live life to the best of their ability, then we need to do it also. This again brings us back to the idea of practising what we preach, and recognizing that the battle is not just about the face-to-face work but all aspects of our role.

Having the freedom to act and practise in a way that suits us and those we help is not a freestanding phenomenon or way of being; most of us need the support of our managers. Although integrity plays a part in being allowed to be the helper we want or need to be, we must also be able to share our vision for the work that is taking place and to educate managers. If we are enthused by the work we do and help we give, then part of our role is to infect others with our enthusiasm and to provide a clear rationale for our activities. In the current climate of targets, numbers and 'special-ized' helping, the focus of managers tends to be different from our own. In order to secure funding and the continuation of services and projects, man-agers have to be able to justify the relevance of the work or helping that takes place. They have tended to become more and more concerned with clearly demonstrable outputs and outcomes. Although a part of this is a numbers game, if our managers feel passionately about what takes place, and have some justification for the approach taken, then they are more likely to go that extra mile in securing the future of a project. Unfortu-nately, managers may have little appreciation of the situations that helpers face, the nature of the work, and of the difficulties of making any honest assessment of outcome (Jeffs and Smith 2005, pp.87–90). The organiza-tional settings in which helpers function, agency priorities, and the expectations managers have of workers are often muddled. This is a dou-ble-edged sword. Workers can exploit this to make more room for more localized and holistic forms of helping, but they are more likely to be left out to dry if things 'go wrong'.

All this poses a difficult question: how do we get our managers to appreciate and understand what they are not part of on a daily basis?

Workers or helpers may shy away from 'the boss' joining in with a session or observing what happens. This may be for a myriad of reasons – some valid, some not – but what we need to consider is that if we don't create room for the helping that happens to be witnessed, it creates an air of mysticism. Shrouding what we do can often alienate people and may cause us to be experienced as a 'forgotten outpost' which may have significance when it comes to allocation or priority of funding. If as helpers we work to include people and enthuse them through participation, then this needs to extend to our managers.

We can return to the work of Parker J. Palmer to explore how we have to be careful of labelling solo working as freedom and ignoring the factor of isolation (1998, p.142). If we close the door of our helping environment to those who may not be directly involved then our work is experienced through evaluation questionnaires and second-hand accounts. These, Palmer argues, cannot capture the nuances of our work, and the only honest way of evaluating the teaching or helping that takes place is to be there and see it for yourself (1998, p.143). This access to our teaching or helping should widen further than just allowing our managers to experience first-hand what we do. We also need to extend the invitation to the community of workers or helpers we are a part of. As helpers we have a wealth of knowledge and experience at our fingertips; we have each other. Using other helpers as a resource can allow us to test out our ideas and use other people's perspectives to develop our ideas and work.

Looking beyond our organizations

Another possibility for helpers who feel constrained by the culture, expectations and requirements of their organization is to develop the work in other settings, or in association with other groups or agencies. There are various options here. One is to use umbrella organizations – especially those that the organization is already associated with. As a worker for example, one of us (Mark) regularly contributed to a grouping of similar agencies to build up projects and initiatives that his employer was uncomfortable with. There were some issues around spending time, and involving people associated with the organization, with such a grouping. However, as the agency was already involved and took advantage of services on offer, there was a degree of room for manoeuvre. Another route taken by a number of the helpers we have talked to is to look to the groups and organizations that they belong to as individuals. Many have looked to their church or religious group as a setting where new work could be developed. Examples included counselling services around discrete areas of interest, community provision, and opportunities for alternative education. In these settings they were working as volunteers. Some employers can be unhappy about this – especially where we are employed in the same area as we volunteer. However, many recognize that this is an area where it can be difficult to find sound grounds for intervention.

A further option lies in the cultivation of new groups and networks – especially where our brief has some development element. Our interest or concern may well have arisen in response to a direct need expressed by people within the community. An example here can be taken from Heather's practice. As a centre-based youth worker Heather's priority was the evening sessions and school holiday activities attended by the local young people. Through interaction with parents of the young people and people within the community, a need was expressed by local parents for a low-key parent and toddler session. Although there were already groups within the community they were more formal (governmental targets featured) and more about the toddlers. What the local mothers wanted was a group where they could find support for themselves as well as the development of their children. With this in mind Heather helped to set up a small group. Integral to the development and realization of the group were two mothers who were able to articulate exactly what was needed from the session. It was Heather's role to create a safe environment for the children and parents and facilitate the 'building' side of the group. The 'helping' that took place within the session was largely between the parents and any more organized activities that took place with the children, such as singing, was directed by the parents. The luxury of not having specified targets and curriculum allowed the creation of space for people to 'be' with each other. Community relationships were also strengthened as many of the parents who attended the group had older children who attended the youth centre. It is important to realize that the helping role in the above example was more about practical facilitation than emotional or personal helping. The aim of developing local spaces is to provide the opportunity for people to come together and realize their own aims. This serves as a tool for people to develop their own frames of reference and often means the project, group or association has life beyond the initial helper.

In addition to the above, another common strategy adopted by helpers is to look for funders that will support their efforts to redirect, deepen and extend their work. Within third sector organizations it is often possible to make the case for taking on the sorts of approaches to helping that we have been exploring here if there are alternative sources of funding and support available. As a result many helpers wanting to work holistically need entre-preneurial qualities. They have to be able to articulate their vision, write project proposals, and find the right trusts and charities to support them. They then have to be able to actually develop the project and the work. It is, perhaps, not surprising that many do not want to take this on – resign-ing themselves to the constraints or simply hoping that someone else will get the money in. Such are the systems that we can find ourselves in, and the perceived costs of standing against them, that we may give up on our ideals. It is sometimes easy to slip into ways of being and working that do little to really help others, or to pretend that somehow our continued par-ticipation is for the best. To be true we either have to fight for work that enhances flourishing or we have to get out.

In a number of situations we may well judge that it is not within our powers – even when acting with others – to make any significant progress toward building a role for the sort of helping we are exploring here. As a result we look to change our job or involvement. Luckily, with continuing social and economic change, and the inability of dominant ideologies and practices to push out alternatives, there are spaces opening up as others are closing down. Unfortunately, though, the openings are not often at the rate or on the scale that we would hope.

Engaging creatively with civil society

Many of the helpers we have been concerned with in this book work within or alongside local organizations, churches and religious groups, and community groups. As we have seen this allows them to access various local networks, and gets them known in an area. It also often provides an orienting framework for their helping that assists more holistic and open forms of helping. Crucially, it can also signal legitimacy for their work. Because they are frequently not locked into state funding and monitoring they are also often viewed more kindly by those seeking help than state-sponsored and provided services. Helpers who want to work holistically, whether or not they are linked into local institutions, we believe, need to be participating and organizing in groups where there is a conscious commitment to engaging with civil society.

Civil society

Like Michael Edwards, we see civil society as simultaneously 'a goal to aim for, a means to achieve it, and a framework for engaging with each-other about ends and means' (Edwards 2005). It is:

> ...essentially *collective* action – in associations, across society and through the public sphere – and as such it provides an essential counterweight to individualism; as *creative* action, civil society provides a much-needed antidote to the cynicism that infects so much of contemporary politics; and as *values-based action*, civil society provides a balance to the otherwise-overbearing influence of state authority and the temptations and incentives of the market, even if those values are contested, as they often are.

While there are various debates around the notion of civil society (and this particular interpretation), we believe it remains a key focus for action – and that there are some obvious social and political reasons for helpers to engage with it.

In the current context where there have been both significant changes brought about by globalization, and a general increase in state surveillance of, and intervention into, people's lives there is a strong case for creating counterbalancing forces. Alessandro Buonfino and Geoff Mulgan (2006, p.4) comment that policymakers have consistently either failed or chosen to ignore 'the webs of informal mutual support that are decisive in helping people to get by, to live, to learn, or be healthy'. They continue in the context of Britain:

> Social science has repeatedly confirmed that small scale – in nations, organizations or places – is associated with stronger bonds. Yet this lesson was repeatedly ignored as structures were scaled up, as professionalism and system were privileged over self-organization, and as expert opinion was given more weight than the views of the public.

Even where there is an attempt to use state power to create a fairer society (for example with regard to the opportunities of different ethnic groups), 'modernisers may be forgetting the importance of informal moral economies in giving ordinary people some power to control their own lives according to their own values: some stake in the system' (Dench, Gavron and Young 2006, p.230).

> Most people in all communities believe in the value of informal mutual support in sustaining a decent and humane society. But the over-centralization of welfare in the name of strict equality is stifling this. Face-to-face relationships carry little weight when confronted by faceless policies from the state. (2006, p.230)

In advocating engagement with civil society and preparedness to step outside normal bureaucratic or organizational structures, we are aware of some of the difficulties that might arise – but the opportunities are significant.

Jazz

As the outpouring of initiatives around the global environmental crisis demonstrates, a philosophy of 'Just do it' – not waiting upon governments and organizations to take action – has brought significant gains. Similarly, community development activity in the United States ranging from health initiatives to public journalism has shown some of the possibilities for civic renewal (Sirianni and Friedland 2001). We believe there is considerable mileage in these developments for thinking about helping. What James Gustave Speth calls 'Jazz' – unscripted, voluntary initiatives that are decentralized and improvisational – can be a significant antidote to the stultifying, 'joined-up' government that both Dench *et al.* and Buonfino and Mulgan allude to.

First, the work that people like Speth (2005) catalogues provides us with various examples of how local initiatives informed by a 'let's do it' philosophy can make a difference. The argument for the contribution of Jazz isn't some Utopian dream, it is based in evidenced practice. One of the particular benefits in terms of helping is that, when we lose some of the bureaucratic and organizational shackles, we can develop much more responsive and engaging ways of working. This has certainly the experience of one us (Mark) in work with local projects associated with the Rank

Foundation over a number of years. The fact that these organizations and groups were not part of a large bureaucracy, did not have to work to externally defined objectives and had some freedom to create an identity that appeals, meant that people sought them out. Furthermore, what they may lack in resources is often more than compensated for by their ability to innovate and develop new forms. Significant social innovation seems to come disproportionately from smaller groups and organizations. Further, the most lasting impacts of such innovation are often not the result of organizational growth. Rather, they come from 'encouraging emulators, and transforming how societies think (with new concepts, arguments and stories)' (Mulgan *et al.* 2007, p.2).

Second, the Jazz model – that of a range of different and often uncoordinated responses and initiatives, often animated and facilitated by third sector or non-governmental organizations and groups – allows for the engagement of civil society (Edwards 2004). It addresses the concerns of many commentators with regard to welfare centralization. As Ann Bookman 2004, p.224) has shown in the United States, new forms of community involvement are taking shape in cities, suburban towns and small rural communities: 'they look different from the PTA volunteerism of the 1950s, but they are no less important to the families involved'. State and other services, indeed democratic processes themselves, are prone to decay and alienation (Mulgan 2007, p.320). They require the stimuli and challenge of 'external' groups, movements and organizations for renewal to take place.

Third, Speth and others, by pointing to the ways in which Jazz can work alongside, and engage with, wider political processes, show some of the ways in which we can begin to transcend some of the either/or dynamics that occur in debates around helping, education and community development. To argue for work that is firmly located in civil society is not to deny the role of the state nor of the private sector. It is simply to recognize, for example, that the more the state intervenes in some key areas of local community life – such as the cultivation of social capital – the more likely it is to destroy what it is seeking to support (Field 2003). But, community-based projects and activities can only go so far though. In Ann Bookman's (2004, p.202) words, they can help to 'mend holes in the fabric of civil society', but full repair (*tikuun olam* in the Jewish tradition) is a much larger project. The problem of the unequal access to resources, systems and capital (of various kinds) remains, and requires sustained political intervention.

There needs to be a shift in the way that we conceptualize and organize education and welfare. We need to grasp the fact that many helping activities are often better when local and grounded in civil society. We also need to take steps ourselves to make things happen. Individual moral courage is the 'seed of radical change' (Mulgan 2007, p.233) but we also need to act with others to change people's experiences of their local communities and networks, of being workers and consumers, and of the state. For helpers this means being part of local networks, participating in their community of practice, and engaging with civil society.

Developing policies to support helping

There are a number of obvious areas where action can be taken to facilitate the development of more holistic approaches to helping others in local organizations, commercial undertakings and state-sponsored services. First and foremost it entails, of course, convincing policymakers and those who control the purse strings of the benefits of supporting helping that is localized, flexible and relational. There are formidable problems around this, but at least there are signs that some politicians are beginning to question dominant approaches. One factor in this has been that, despite substantially increased levels of funding in countries like the UK, services have not improved standards at the rate expected (see, for example, Wanless, Appleby and Harrison (2007) on health service reform). While a radical shift in approach is unlikely in the short term, there is always the possibility of pockets of freer funding that can be exploited by alert agencies and groups. In addition to this, at the level of local state services, there have been some indicators of a growing internal dissatisfaction with current ways of working. The move into children's services in England, for example, has led to some initiatives where social workers are able to work more on their own initiative – but, unfortunately, the same outcome framework remains (O'Hara 2007). It may well be that some local workers and managers within state services will be able to exploit gaps to facilitate more creative and satisfying approaches. However, any significant advance requires reversing the centralization and bureaucratization of welfare; reducing the focus on targets and upon demonstrating short-term outcomes; and the abandoning of inappropriate models and ways of thinking drawn from the commercial sector.

In the meantime it is worth thinking about the sorts of arrangements and priorities that will be necessary if helping of the kind we have been discussing is to flourish with state involvement. Here three particular things recommend themselves. First, there is a clear need for autonomous arenas of practice within key institutions such as schools, colleges, and housing services and associations. Within schools, for example, there is evidence of a growing need for spaces for reflection and exploration for young people where there is no requirement to link into the standard reporting and record-keeping systems. To some extent this has been recognized within the Scottish community schools initiative – but the solution has been simply to report to a different arm of the state. Second, there needs to be a major rethink around the way third sector and civil society organizations and groups are supported by the state. Many current funding arrangements turn groups and organizations into an annex of the state – leaving little degree of discretion for frontline workers (Leather 2007; NCVO 2007). Instead there should be a return to seconding helpers to local groups and agencies; and an exploration of new forms of grant-giving rather than service-level agreements and the like. Third, systems and policies need to be reworked so that short-term and more improvisational initiatives can be supported and worked alongside – and social innovations generated.

Conclusion

We have been examining a form of helping that involves listening and exploring issues and problems with people; and teaching and giving advice; and providing direct assistance; and where helpers are local and seen as people of integrity. We have also argued for a move beyond ways of working currently prized as 'professional' to embrace more local and improvisational helping. This way of understanding helping may well strike a chord with many working in religious organizations, local groups and social movements. However, where we enter more bureaucratic arenas helping tends to be stripped of much of its moral dimension and utility. It also loses touch with a great deal of the supporting language and thinking. Words like boundary, client, delivery, intervention and outcome replace the discourse of friendship, association, relationship and faith. All this can be seen as a move from a concern with practical wisdom and the desire to act truly and rightly (what Aristotle talks about as *phronesis*) to a focus on what is correct (according to bureaucratic rules) and technique (*techne*). Luckily significant spaces remain where helpers can remain true to their calling. Bureaucratic professionalism may well be working itself into a corner. We hope more will have the courage and opportunity to develop spaces where helping is on a human scale; and where there are people who are able to be around and there for others, and around whom wisdom flourishes.

Further reading and web support

- Bok, S. (1999) *Lying: Moral Choice in Public and Private Life.* New York, NY: Vintage. Bok's book has become the central modern treatment of lying and repays careful reading.

- Ginsborg, P. (2005) *The Politics of Everyday Life: Making Choices, Changing Lives.* New Haven, CT: Yale University Press. This is a helpful diagnosis of the problems of representative democracies and exploration of the possibilities of local civic action.

- Mulgan, G. (2007) *Good and Bad Power: The Ideals and Betrayals of Government.* London: Penguin. This is an interesting exploration of the democratic state and why renewal and challenge are so important.

- Speth, J.G. (2005) *Red Sky at Morning: America and the Crisis of the Global Environment.* New Haven, CT: Yale University Press. 'Just doing it' – not waiting upon national governments and international organizations to take action – has led to a remarkable outpouring of initiatives around the global environmental crisis. However, James Gustave Speth's vision of unscripted, voluntary initiatives that are decentralized and improvisational – what he calls 'Jazz' – has considerable potential for thinking about what we do as helpers.

For further discussion of the ideas explored in this chapter, suggestions for further reading and links to other sources, go to our support page at: www.infed.org/helping/getting_from_here_to_there.htm

Bibliography

Allen, D. (2001) *Getting Things Done: How to Achieve Stress-free Productivity.* London: Piatkus.

Arendt, H. (1959) *The Human Condition.* New York, NY: Doubleday/Anchor.

Aristotle (1987) *The Nicomachean Ethics* (trans. J. E. C. Welldon). Amherst, MA: Prometheus Books.

Arnold, M. (1993) *'Culture and Anarchy' and Other Writings,* ed. S. Colloni. Cambridge: Cambridge University Press.

Avnon, D. (1998) *Martin Buber: The Hidden Dialogue.* Lanham, MD: Rowman and Littlefield.

Barton, D. and Tusting, K. (eds) (2005) *Beyond Communities of Practice: Language Power and Social Context.* Cambridge: Cambridge University Press.

Beem, C. (1999) *The Necessity of Politics: Reclaiming American Public Life.* Chicago, IL: University of Chicago Press.

Bekerman, Z., Burbules, N. C. and Keller, D. S. (2006) *Learning in Places: The Informal Education Reader.* New York, NY: Peter Lang.

Bellah, R. N., Madsen, R., Sullivan, W. M., Swidler, A. and Tipton, S. M. (1996) *Habits of the Heart: Individualism and Commitment in American Life,* 2nd ed. Berkeley, CA: University of California Press.

Bernstein, R. R. J. (1983) *Beyond Objectivism and Relativism: Science, Hermeneutics and Praxis.* Oxford: Blackwell.

Biestek, F. P. (1961) *The Casework Relationship.* London: Unwin University Books.

Bishop, J. and Hoggett, P. (1986) *Organizing Around Enthusiasms: Mutual Aid in Leisure.* London: Comedia.

Blackburn, S. (2005) *Truth: A Guide for the Perplexed.* London: Allen Lane.

Board of Education (1944) *Teachers and Youth Leaders. Report of the Committee appointed by the President of the Board of Education to consider the supply, recruitment and training of teachers and youth leaders.* London: HMSO. Part 2 available at www.infed.org/archives/e-texts/mcnair_part_two.htm, accessed 5 February 2008.

Bok, S. (1999) *Lying: Moral Choice in Public and Private Life,* 2nd ed. New York, NY: Vintage Books.

Bolton, G. (2005) *Reflective Practice: Writing and Professional Development.* London: Sage.

Bookman, A. (2004) *Starting in Our Own Backyards: How Working Families Can Build Community and Survive the New Economy.* New York, NY: Routledge.

Boud, D., Keogh, R. and Walker, D. (eds) (1985) *Reflection: Turning Experience into Learning.* London: Kogan Page.

Brackett, J. R. (1904) *Supervision and Education in Charity.* New York, NY: Macmillan.

Brandon, D. (1990) *Zen in the Art of Helping.* London: Penguin Arkana. First published 1976, London: Routledge & Kegan Paul.

Brew, J. M. (1943) *In the Service of Youth.* London: Faber & Faber.

Brew, J. M. (1946) *Informal Education: Adventures and Reflections.* London: Faber & Faber.

Brew, J. M. (1957) *Youth and Youth Groups.* London: Faber and Faber.

Briggs, L. L. (2004) *The Art of Helping: What to Say and Do When Someone Is Hurting.* Colorado Springs, CO: River Oak Publishing.

Brinton, H. H. (1972) *Quaker Journals: Varieties of Religious Experience Among Friends.* Wallingford, PA: Pendle Hill Publications.

Brown, A. (1986) *Modern Political Philosophy: Theories of the Just Society.* Harmondsworth: Penguin.

Buber, M. (1947) *Between Man and Man.* London: Kegan Paul. New edition 2002, London: Routledge.

Buber, M. (1958) *I and Thou,* 2nd ed. (Transl. R. Gregory Smith). Edinburgh: T. & T. Clark.

Buonfino, A., and Mulgan, G. (2006) 'Introduction.' In A. Buonfino and Geoff Mulgan (eds) *Porcupines in Winter: The Pleasures and Pains of Living Together in Modern Britain.* London: The Young Foundation.

Carkoff, R. R. (2000) *The Art of Helping in the 21st Century,* 8th ed. Amherst, MA: Human Resource Development Press.

Casement, P. (1985) *On Learning from the Patient.* London: Routledge.

Chara, P. J. (1999) *The Art of Virtue.* Enumclaw, WA: Wine Press Publishing.

Cohen, D. and Prusak, L. (2001) *In Good Company: How Social Capital Makes Organizations Work.* Boston, MA: Harvard Business School Press.

Colley, H. (2003) *Mentoring for Social Inclusion: A Critical Approach to Nurturing Mentor Relationships.* London: RoutledgeFalmer.

Collins, M. (1991) *Adult Education as Vocation: A Critical Role for the Adult Educator.* London: Routledge.

Comte-Sponville, A. (2001) *A Short Treatise on the Great Virtues: The Use of Philosophy in Everyday Life.* London: William Heinemann.

Crisp, R. and Slote, M. (1997) *Virtue Ethics.* Oxford: Oxford University Press.

Crosby, M. (2001) 'Working with People as an Informal Educator.' In L. D. Richardson and M. Wolfe (eds) *Principles and Practice of Informal Education: Learning Through Life.* London: RoutledgeFalmer.

Culley, S. and Bond, T. (2004) *Integrative Counselling Skills in Action*, 2nd ed. London: Sage.

Davies, B. D. and Gibson, A. (1967) *The Social Education of the Adolescent*. London: University of London Press.

Dawson, J. B. (1926) 'The casework supervisor in a family agency,' *Family 6*, 293–95.

de Tocqueville, A.(1994) *Democracy in America*. London: Fontana.

Dench, G., Gavron, K. and Young, M. (2006) *The New East End: Kinship, Race and Conflict*. London: Profile Books.

Dewey, J. (1933) *How We Think*. New York, NY: D. C. Heath.

Doyle, M. E. (1999) 'Called to be an informal educator.' In *Youth and Policy 65*, autumn, 28–37. Also available at www.infed.org/christianeducation/calling-doyle.htm, accessed 5 February 2008.

Duck, S. (1999) *Relating to Others*, 2nd ed. Buckingham: Open University Press.

Edwards, M. (2004) *Civil Society*. Cambridge: Polity.

Edwards, M. (2005) *Civil Society*. Available at www.infed.org/association/civil_society.htm, accessed 5 February 2008.

Egan, G. (2002, 2006) *The Skilled Helper: A Problem-management and Opportunity-development Approach to Helping*, 7th and 8th eds. Belmont, CA: Thomson/Brooks Cole.

Eisner, E. W. (1985) *The Art of Educational Evaluation: A Personal View*. London: Falmer Press.

Eisner, E. W. (1998) *The Enlightened Eye: Qualitative Inquiry and the Enhancement of Educational Practice*. Upper Saddle River, NJ: Merrill.

Eisner, E. W. (2002) *What can Education Learn from the Arts about the Practice of Education?* Available at www.infed.org/biblio/eisner_arts_and_the_practice_of_education.htm, accessed 5 February 2008.

Elsdon, K. T. with Reynolds, J. and Stewart, S. (1995) *Voluntary Organizations: Citizenship, Learning and Change*. Leicester: NIACE.

Field, J. (2003) *Social Capital*. London: Routledge.

Foster, R.J. (1998) *Celebration of Discipline: The Path to Spiritual Growth*. New York, NY: HarperCollins.

Fox, G. (1998) *The Journal*, ed. Nigel Smith. London: Penguin.

Freire, P. (1972) *Pedagogy of the Oppressed*. Harmondsworth: Penguin.

Freud, S. (1973) *Introducing Lectures on Psychoanalysis*. Harmondsworth: Penguin.

Fromm, E. (1979) *To Have or To Be*. London: Abacus. (First published 1976).

Fromm, E. (1995) *The Art of Loving*. London: Thorsons. (First published 1957).

Fullinwider, R. K. (2007) *Sissela Bok on Lying and Moral Choice in Private and Public Life: an Amplification*. Available at www.infed.org/thinkers/bok_lying.htm, accessed 5 February 2008.

Gadamer, H-G. (1979) *Truth and Method*, 2nd ed. London: Sheed and Ward.

Garrett, P. M. (2005) 'Social work's "electronic turn": notes on the deployment of information and communication technologies in social work with children and families.' *Critical Social Policy 25*, 4, 529–53.

Geldard, K. and Geldard, D. (2004) *Counselling Adolescents*, 2nd ed. London: Sage.

Gilman, J. E. (2001) *Fidelity of the Heart: An Ethic of Christian Virtue.* New York, NY: Oxford University Press.

Gilroy, P. (1987) *There Ain't No Black in the Union Jack: The Cultural Politics of Race and Nation.* London: Hutchinson.

Ginsborg, P. (2005) *The Politics of Everyday Life: Making Choices, Changing Lives.* New Haven, CT: Yale University Press.

Goetschius, G. W. and Tash, M. J. (1967) *Working with Unattached Youth: Problem, Approach, Method.* London: Routledge & Kegan Paul.

Goffman, E. (1963) *Behavior in Public Places: Notes on the Social Organization of Gatherings.* New York, NY: Free Press of Glencoe.

Guignon, C.(2004) *On Being Authentic.* London: Routledge.

Guillory, J. (1995) *Cultural Capital: The Problem of Literary Canon Formation.* Chicago, IL: University of Chicago Press.

Haber, J. G. (ed) (1993) *Doing and Being: Selected Readings in Moral Philosophy.* New York, NY: Macmillan.

Habermas, J. (1984) *The Theory of Communicative Action. Vol. 1: Reason and the Rationalization of Society* (trans. T. McCarthy). Cambridge: Polity Press.

Haidt, J. (2006) *Happiness Hypothesis: Putting Ancient Wisdom to the Test of Modern Science.* London: William Heinemann.

Halpin, D. (2003) *Hope and Education: The Role of the Utopian Imagination.* London: RoutledgeFalmer.

Hartley, J. (2001) *Reading Groups.* Oxford: Oxford University Press.

Harvey, J. (2006) *Valuing and Educating Young People: Stern Love the Lyward Way.* London: Jessica Kingsley Publishers.

Havinghurst, R. J. (1972) *Developmental Tasks and Education*, 3rd ed. New York, NY: D. McKay.

Hirsch, B. J. (2005) *A Place to Call Home: After-school Programs for Urban Youth.* New York, NY: Teachers College Press.

HM Government (2004) *Every Child Matters: Change for Children.* London: Department for Education and Skills.

Hodes, A. (1975) *Encounter with Martin Buber.* Harmondsworth: Penguin.

Hodgkin, R. (1991) 'Michael Polanyi: Prophet of life, the universe and everything.' *Times Higher Educational Supplement*, 27 September, 15.

Holly, M. L. (1989) *Writing to Grow: Keeping a Personal-professional Journal.* Portsmouth, NH: Heinemann.

hooks, b. (2003) *Teaching Community: A Pedagogy of Hope.* New York, NY: Routledge.

Houle, C.(1980) *Continuing Learning in the Professions.* San Francisco, CA: Jossey-Bass.

Howe, D. (1993) *On Being a Client: Understanding the Process of Counselling in Psychotherapy.* London: Sage.

Hursthouse, R. (1999) *On Virtue Ethics.* Oxford: Oxford University Press.

James, O. (2007) *Affluenza: How to be Successful and Stay Sane.* London: Vermillion.

Jeffs, T. (2006) *Too Few, Too Many: The Retreat from Vocation and Calling.* Available at www.infed.org/talkingpoint/retreat_from_calling_and_vocation.htm, accessed 5 February 2008.

Jeffs, T. and Smith, M. K. (eds) (1990) *Using Informal Education.* Buckingham: Open University Press.

Jeffs, T. and Smith, M. K. (2005) *Informal Education: Conversation, Democracy and Learning,* 3rd ed. Nottingham: Educational Heretics Press.

Jeffs, T. and Smith, M. K. (2006) 'Where is *Youth Matters* taking us?' *Youth and Policy 91,* 23–39.

Johns, C. (2004) *Becoming a Reflective Practitioner.* Oxford: Blackwell.

Kadushin, A. and Harness, D. (2002) *Supervision in Social Work,* 4th ed. New York, NY: Columbia University Press.

Kane, J. (2003) *How to Heal: A Guide for Caregivers.* New York, NY: Helios Press.

Kearney, R. (2003) *Strangers, Gods and Monsters: Interpreting Otherness.* London: Routledge.

Kekes, J. (1995) *Moral Wisdom and Good Lives.* Ithaca, NY: Cornell University Press.

Kirkman, R. L. (1992) *Theories of Truth: A Critical Introduction.* Cambridge, MA: MIT Press.

Kirschenbaum, H. and Henderson, V. L. (eds) (1990) *The Carl Rogers Reader.* London: Constable.

Klug, R. (2002) *How to Keep a Spiritual Journal: A Guide to Journal Keeping for Inner Growth and Personal Discovery,* rev. ed. Minneapolis, MN: Augsburg.

Kolb, D. A. (1984) *Experiential Learning.* Englewood Cliffs, NJ: Prentice-Hall.

Kottler, J. A. (2000) *Doing Good: Passion and Commitment for Helping Others.* New York, NY: Brunner-Routledge.

Kraemer, K. (2003) *Martin Buber's "I and Thou": Practicing Living Dialogue.* New York, NY: Paulist Press International.

Lane, R. E. (2000) *The Loss of Happiness in Market Economies.* New Haven, CT: Yale University Press.

Lave, J. and Wenger, E. (1991) *Situated Learning: Legitimate Peripheral Participation.* Cambridge: Cambridge University Press.

Layard, R. (2005) *Happiness: Lessons from a New Science.* London: Allen Lane.

Layder, D. R. (2004) *Social and Personal Identity: Understanding Your Self.* London: Sage.

Leather, S. (2007) *Speech to the NCVO Annual Conference, 21 February 2007.* Charity Commission. Available at www.charity-commission.gov.uk/recent_changes/speech.asp, accessed 5 February 2008

London Edinburgh Weekend Return Group (working group of the Conference of Socialist Economists) (1980) *In and Against the State.* London: Pluto Press.

Lykken, D. T. (1999) *Happiness: The Nature and Nurture of Joy and Contentment.* New York, NY: St Martin's Press.

Macpherson, C. B. (1962) *The Political Theory of Possessive Individualism.* Oxford: Oxford University Press.

MacIntyre, A. (1985) *After Virtue: A Study in Moral Theory.* London: Duckworth.

Marsella, A. J., Devos, G. and Hsu, F. L. K. (eds) (1985) *Culture and Self: Asian and Western Perspectives.* London: Tavistock.

Martin, P. (2005) *Making Happy People: The Nature of Happiness and its Origins in Childhood.* London: Fourth Estate.

McLaughlin, M. W., Irby, M. A. and Langman, J. (1994) *Urban Sanctuaries: Neighborhood Organizations in the Lives and Futures of Inner-city Youth.* San Francisco, CA: Jossey-Bass.

McLeod, J. (2003) *An Introduction to Counselling,* 3rd ed. Maidenhead: Open University Press.

Mills, C. W.(1959) *The Sociological Imagination.* New York, NY: Oxford University Press.

Mills, C. W. (1963) 'The Professional Ideology of Social Pathologists.' In I. L. Horowitz (ed.) *Power, Politics and People: The Collected Essays of C. Wright Mills.* New York, NY: Oxford University Press. (First published in 1943 in the *American Journal of Sociology 49,* 2).

Milson, F. (1968) *Growing with the Job: Youth Worker's Progress.* London: National Association of Youth Clubs. Available at www.infed.org/archives/nayc/milson_growing.htm, accessed 5 February 2008.

Mitchell, .T. (2006) *Michael Polanyi: The Art of Knowing.* Wilmington, DE: Intercollegiate Studies Institute.

Moon, J. A. (1999) *Reflection in Learning and Professional Development: Theory and Practice.* London: RoutledgeFalmer.

Mulgan, G. (2007) *Good and Bad Power: The Ideals and Betrayals of Government.* London: Penguin.

Mulgan, G., with Rushanara, A., Halkett, R. and Sanders, B. (2007) *In and Out of Sync: The Challenge of Growing Social Innovations.* London: National Endowment for Science, Technology and the Arts.

Newman, M. (2006) *Teaching Defiance: Stories and Strategies for Activist Educators.* San Francisco, CA: Jossey-Bass.

NCVO (National Council of Voluntary Organizations) (2007) *The UK Voluntary Sector Almanac 2007.* London: NCVO.

Noddings, N. (1992) *The Challenge to Care in Schools.* New York, NY: Teachers College Press.

Noddings, N. (2002) *Starting at Home: Caring and Social Policy.* Berkeley, CA: University of California Press.

Noddings, N. (2003a) *Happiness and Education*. New York, NY: Cambridge University Press.

Noddings, N. (2003b) *Caring: A Feminine Approach to Ethics and Moral Education*, 2nd ed. Berkeley, CA: University of California Press.

Noddings, N. (2005) *Caring in education*. Available at www.infed.org/biblio/ noddings_caring_in_education.htm, accessed 5 February 2008.

Offer, A. (2006) *The Challenge of Affluence: Self-control and Well-being in the United States and Britain since 1950*. Oxford: Oxford University Press.

O'Hara, M. (2007) *Change of Culture*. The Guardian – Society, 1 August. Available at http://society.guardian.co.uk/careers/story/0,,2138639,00.html, accessed 5 February 2008.

Ord, J. (2004) 'The youth work curriculum and the Transforming Youth Work agenda,' *Youth and Policy 83*, 43–59.

Oriah Mountain Dreamer (2000) *The Invitation*. London: Thorsons.

Page, S. and Wosket, V. (1994) *Supervising the Counsellor: A Cyclical Model*. London: Routledge.

Pahl, R. (2000) *On Friendship*. Cambridge: Polity Press.

Palmer, P. J. (1983, 1993) *To Know as We are Known: Education as a Spiritual Journey*. San Francisco, CA: Harper.

Palmer, P. J. (1997) 'The grace of great things: recovering the sacred in knowing, teaching, and learning.' *Spirituality in Education*. Available at www.couragerenewal.org/resources/writings/grace, accessed 5 February 2008.

Palmer, P. J. (1998) *The Courage to Teach: Exploring the Inner Landscape of a Teacher's Life*. San Francisco, CA: Jossey-Bass.

Palmer, P. J. (2000) *Let Your Life Speak*. San Francisco, CA: Jossey-Bass.

Perlman, H. H. (1979) *Relationship: The Heart of Helping People*. Chicago, IL: University of Chicago Press.

Peters, D. E. (1967) *Supervision in Social Work: A Method of Student Training and Staff Development*. London: George Allen & Unwin.

Polanyi, M. (1958, 1998) *Personal Knowledge: Towards a Post Critical Philosophy*. London: Routledge.

Polanyi, M. (1967) *The Tacit Dimension*. New York, NY: Anchor Books.

Pope, Alexander (1994) '*Essay on Man' and Other Essays*. Mineola, NY: Dover. Also downloadable from Project Gutenberg at www.gutenberg.org/etext/2428, accessed 5 February 2008.

Prochaska, F. (2006) *Christianity and Social Service in Modern Britain: The Disinherited Spirit*. Oxford: Oxford University Press.

Progoff, I. (1975) *At a Journal Workshop*. New York, NY: Dialogue House Library.

Punshon, J. (1984) *Portrait in Grey: A Short History of the Quakers*. London: Quaker Home Service.

Punshon, J. (1987) *Encounter with Silence: Reflections from the Quaker Tradition.* Richmond, IN: Friends United Press.

Putnam, R. D. (2000) *Bowling Alone: The Collapse and Revival of American Community.* New York, NY: Simon and Schuster.

Rainer, T. (2004) *The New Diary: How to Use a Journal for Self-guidance and Extended Creativity.* Los Angeles, CA: J. P. Tarcher Inc.

Reid, K. E. (1981) 'Formulation of a method, 1920–1936' in *From Character Building to Social Treatment: The History of the Use of Groups in Social Work.* Westport, CT. Available at www.infed.org/archives/e-texts/reid_groupwork_formulation_method.htm, accessed 6 February 2008.

Rhodes. J. E. (2002) *Stand by Me: The Risks and Rewards of Mentoring Today's Youth.* Cambridge, MA: Harvard University Press.

Richardson, L. (2000) 'Writing: A Method of Inquiry.' In N. K. Denzin and Yvonna S. Lincoln (eds) *Handbook of Qualitative Research,* 2nd ed. London: Sage.

Richmond, M. E. (1899) *Friendly Visiting Among the Poor: A Handbook for Charity Workers.* New York, NY: Macmillan.

Richmond, M. E. (1917) *Social Diagnosis.* New York, NY: Russell Sage Foundation.

Richmond, M. E. (1922) *What is Social Case Work? An Introductory Description.* New York, NY: Russell Sage Foundation.

Ridley, M. (1997) *The Origins of Virtue.* London: Penguin.

Rogers, A. (ed.) (2003) *Inside Youth Work: Insights into Informal Education from Projects Supported by the Rank Foundation and Joseph Rank Trust.* London: Rank Foundation/YMCA George Williams College. Available at www.ymca.ac.uk/rank/publications/inside_youth_work.pdf, accessed 6 February 2008.

Rogers, A. and Smith, M. K. (2006) *Evaluation: Learning What Matters – Conference Workbook.* London: Rank Foundation/YMCA George Williams College. Available at www.ymca.ac.uk/rank/conference/evaluation_learninng_what_matters.pdf, accessed 5 March 2008.

Rogers, C. (1961) *On Becoming a Person: A Therapist's View of Psychotherapy.* Boston, MA: Houghton Mifflin.

Rogers, C. (1967) 'The Interpersonal Relationship in the Facilitation of Learning.' Reprinted in H. Kirschenbaum and V. Land Henderson (eds) (1990) *The Carl Rogers Reader.* London: Constable.

Rogers, C. (1980) *A Way of Being.* Boston, MA: Houghton Mifflin.

Rogers, C. (1990) *The Carl Rogers Reader,* ed. H. Kirschenbaum and V. Land Henderson. London: Constable & Robinson.

Rose, J. (2002) *The Intellectual Life of the British Working Classes.* New Haven, CT: Yale Nota Bene.

Ross, A. (2003) *Counselling Skills for Church and Faith Workers.* Maidenhead: Open University Press.

Roth, J. K. (1995) *International Encyclopaedia of Ethics.* London: Fitzroy Dearborn Publishers.

Salzberger-Wittenberg, I., Henry, G. and Osborne, E. (1983) *The Emotional Experience of Learning and Teaching.* London: Routledge & Kegan Paul.

Sampson, E. E. (1993) *Celebrating the Other: A Dialogic Account of Human Nature.* Hemel Hempstead: Harvester/Wheatsheaf.

Sawyer, P. R. (2005) *Socialization to Civil Society: A Life History of Community Leaders.* New York, NY: Suny Press.

Schön, D. (1983) *The Reflective Practitioner: How Professionals Think in Action.* London: Temple Smith.

Schön, D. (1987) *Educating the Reflective Practitioner.* San Francisco, CA: Jossey-Bass.

Seligman, M. (2003) *Authentic Happiness: Using the New Positive Psychology to Realise Your Potential for Lasting Fulfilment.* London: Nicholas Brealey Publishing.

Shah, H. and Marks, N. (2004) *A Well-being Manifesto for a Flourishing Society.* London: New Economics Foundation. Available at www.neweconomics.org/gen/ z_sys_publicationdetail.aspx?pid=193, accessed 6 February 2008

Sirianni, C. and Friedland, L. (2001) *Civic Innovation in America: Community Empowerment, Public Policy and the Movement for Civic Renewal.* Berkeley, CA: University of California Press.

Smith, H. (2005) 'The year of the volunteer: formalizing the goodwill mountain.' *Youth and Policy 89*, 84–93.

Smith, M. K. (1984) *Questions for Survival: Some Problems of Political Education.* Leicester: NAYC Publications.

Smith, M. K. (1994) *Local Education: Community, Conversation, Praxis.* Buckingham: Open University Press.

Smith, M. K. (1995) 'Developing critical conversations about practice.' *Groupwork 8*, 134–51. Available at www.infed.org/archives/jeffs_and_smith/smith_critical_ conversations.htm, accessed 6 February 2008.

Smith, M. K. (1997, 2005) *The Functions of Supervision.* Available at www.infed.org/biblio/functions_of_supervision.htm, accessed 6 February 2008.

Smith, M. K. (1999, 2006) *Keeping a Learning Journal.* Available at www.infed.org/research/keeping_a_journal.htm, accessed 6 February 2008

Smith, M. K. (2003) *Communities of Practice.* Available at www.infed.org/biblio/communities_of_pratice.htm, accessed 6 February 2008

Smith, M. K. (2006) *Evaluation.* Available at www.infed.org/biblio/b-eval.htm, accessed 6 February 2008

Smith, M. K. (2007) *Classic Studies in Informal Education: Working with Unattached Youth.* Available at www.infed.org/research/working_with_unattached_youth.htm, accessed 6 February 2008

Smith, M. K. and Smith, Michele E. (2002) *Friendship and Informal Education.* Available at www.infed.org/biblio/friendship_and_education.htm, accessed 6 February 2008

Sorabji, R. (2006) *Self: Ancient and Modern Insights about Individuality, Life, and Death.* Oxford: University of Oxford Press.

Speth, J. G. (2005) *Red Sky at Morning: America and the Crisis of the Global Environment.* New Haven, CT: Yale University Press.

Steiner, G. (2003) *Lessons of the Masters: The Charles Eliot Norton Lectures 2001–2002.* Cambridge, MA: Harvard University Press.

Stone, D., Patton, B. and Heen, S. (2000) *Difficult Conversations: How to Discuss What Matters Most.* London: Penguin.

Storkey, E. (1995) *The Search for Intimacy.* London: Hodder & Stoughton.

Taylor, B. (2006) *Reflective Practice: A Guide for Nurses and Midwives,* 2nd ed. Maidenhead: Open University Press.

Taylor, C. (1989) *Sources of the Self: The Making of the Modern Identity.* Cambridge: Cambridge University Press.

Taylor, C. (1991) *The Ethics of Authenticity.* Cambridge, MA: Harvard University Press.

Tennant, M. (1997) *Psychology and Adult Learning.* London: Routledge.

Usher, R. Bryant, I. and Johnston, R. (1997) *Adult Education and the Postmodern Challenge.* London: Routledge.

Vangelisti, A.L. and Perlman, D. (eds) (2006) *The Cambridge Handbook of Personal Relationships.* New York, NY: Cambridge University Press.

Vermes, P.(1988) *Buber.* London: Peter Halban.

Vernon, M. (2007) *The Philosophy of Friendship.* Basingstoke: Palgrave.

Walzer, M. (1997) *On Tolerance.* New Haven, CT: Yale University Press.

Wanless, D., Appleby, J. and Harrison, A. (2007) *Our Future Health Secured? A Review of NHS Funding and Performance.* London: King's Fund. Available at www.kingsfund.org.uk/publications/kings_fund_publications/our_future.html, accessed 6 February 2008

Wenger, E. (1998) 'Communities of practice: learning as a social system.' *Systems Thinker.* Available at www.co-i-l.com/coil/knowledge-garden/cop/lss.shtml, accessed 6 February 2008

Wenger, E. (1999) *Communities of Practice: Learning, Meaning and Identity.* Cambridge: Cambridge University Press.

Whyte, D. (1999) *The Heart Aroused: Poetry and the Preservation of the Soul at Work.* London: The Industrial Society.

Williams, B. (2003) *Truth and Truthfulness: An Essay in Genealogy.* Princeton, NJ: Princeton University Press.

Winnicott, D. W. (1965) *The Maturation Process and the Facilitating Environment.* London: Hogarth Press.

Wolf, A. (2002) *Does Education Matter: Myths About Education and Economic Growth.* London: Penguin.

Woods, P. and Jeffrey, B. (1996) *Teachable Moments: The Art of Teaching in Primary Schools.* Buckingham: Open University Press.

Young, K. (1999) 'The Youth Worker as Guide, Philosopher and Friend.' In S. Banks (ed.) *Ethical Issues in Youth Work.* London: Routledge.

Young, M. E. (1998) *Learning the Art of Helping: Building Blocks and Techniques,* 3rd ed. Upper Saddle River, NJ: Prentice-Hall.

Younghusband, E. (1947) *Report on the Employment and Training of Social Workers.* London: Carnegie United Kingdom Trust.

Subject Index

acceptance, of others 36
access, unequal 151–2
accountability 143
action, encouraging 104–8
actions
   conscious 29
   not imposing 20
activity, shared 14
acts, creative 65
advice, giving appropriately 37
affection 89
affiliation, biochemical base 73
after-school programmes 137
agencies, developing relationships 144–6
agendas, in helping conversation 97–8
agent 29–30
aims, in helping conversation 97–8
aliveness 17
anxiety 21
apprenticeship 126–7
approachability 17–18
arete 27
Aristotle 27–8, 30, 32, 58, 60, 63, 86–7
artful doing 15
artistry 15, 67
assistance, practical 19
attachment 89
attending 99
authenticity 25, 26, 48–50, 55, 102, 142,
   144–5
authority 25, 134, 135
availability 88

balance 29, 88, 113, 118–20
Behavior in Public Places 135
behaviour
   pro-social 30
   and relationships 72–4
being

around 17–18
connected 38–9, 40
discerning 65–7
and having 16–17, 76
knowledgeable 63–5
there 18–19
valued 63
wise 19
with 20
belief systems 47–8
Biestek, Felix 82–3, 86
body idiom 135
boundaries 89–90, 141
Buber, Martin 76–8, 81, 84
Buddhism, virtue 28
bureaucracy 23, 25, 58, 144

calling 23, 54–5
care 23, 54–5
caring 15, 33–8
catching the moment 18
categorization 16
caution, culture of 139
centralization 136
change
   committing to 105–7
   planning 107–8
   system 138–9
character 26, 47–8
characteristics, key 22–3
child abuse 81
child development 74
child protection 34
children, love 28
Christianity, virtue 28
civic model, of community 95
civil society 117, 148–52
client-centred therapy 37–8
coercion 107

Author Index